MACPAC

Medicaid and CHIP Payment and Access Commission

The Medicaid and CHIP Payment and Access Commission (MACPAC) was established in the Children's Health Insurance Program Reauthorization Act of 2009 (CHIPRA) and its charge was later revised in the Patient Protection and Affordable Care Act of 2010. The U.S. Comptroller General appointed 17 Commissioners in December 2009 who have broad perspectives on Medicaid and CHIP drawn from diverse backgrounds and regions of the United States.

The Commission is a non-partisan, federal, analytic support agency and resource for the Congress on Medicaid and CHIP. MACPAC is the first federal agency charged with providing policy and data analysis to the Congress on Medicaid and CHIP, and for making recommendations to the Congress and the Secretary of the Department of Health and Human Services on a wide range of issues affecting these programs. The Commission conducts independent policy analysis and health services research on key Medicaid and CHIP topics, including but not limited to:

- Eligibility, enrollment and benefits;
- Payment;
- Access to care;
- Quality of care;
- Interactions between Medicaid and Medicare; and
- Data development to support policy analysis and program accountability.

As required in its statutory charge, the Commission will submit reports to the Congress on March 15 and June 15 of each year. As applicable, each member of the Commission will vote on recommendations contained in the reports. The reports provide the Congress with a better understanding of the Medicaid and CHIP programs, their roles in the U.S. health care system, and the key policy and data issues to be addressed to guide policies outlined in the Commission's statutory charge.

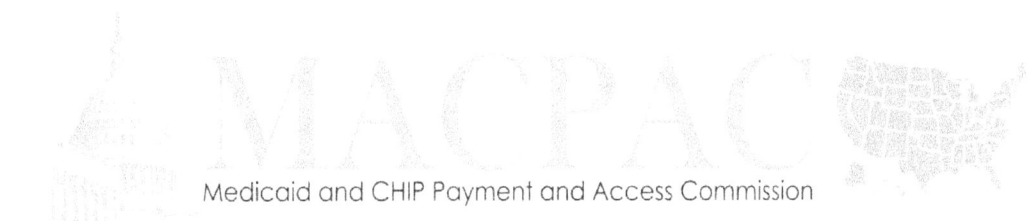

Medicaid and CHIP Payment and Access Commission

Report to the Congress

The Evolution of Managed Care in Medicaid

June 2011

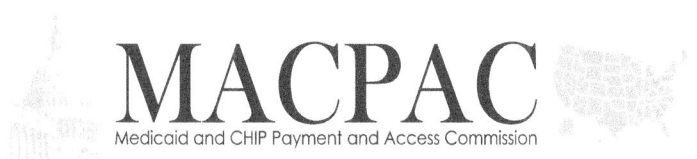

MACPAC
Medicaid and CHIP Payment and Access Commission

1800 M Street, NW
Suite 350 N
Washington, DC 20036
Phone: (202) 273-2460
Fax: (202) 273-2452
www.macpac.gov

Commissioners

Diane Rowland, ScD,
  Chair
David Sundwall, MD,
  Vice Chair

Sharon Carte, MHS
Richard Chambers
Donna Checkett, MPA,
  MSW
Andrea Cohen, JD
Burton Edelstein, DDS,
  MPH
Patricia Gabow, MD
Herman Gray, MD, MBA
Denise Henning, CNM,
  MSN
Mark Hoyt, FSA, MAAA
Norma Martinez Rogers,
  PhD, RN, FAAN
Judith Moore
Trish Riley, MS
Sara Rosenbaum, JD
Robin Smith
Steven Waldren, MD, MS

Lu Zawistowich, ScD,
  Executive Director

June 15, 2011

The Honorable Joseph R. Biden
President of the Senate
U.S. Capitol
Washington, DC 20510

The Honorable John A. Boehner
Speaker of the House
U.S. House of Representatives
U.S. Capitol
H-232
Washington, DC 20515

Dear Mr. Vice President and Mr. Speaker:

It is with great pleasure that, on behalf of the Commission, I submit the Medicaid and CHIP Payment and Access Commission's (MACPAC's) June 2011 *Report to the Congress: The Evolution of Managed Care in Medicaid.* This Report examines managed care in Medicaid, focusing on the enrollees served, participating plans, spending, payment, access, data, and program accountability. This Report builds upon our March 2011 *Report to the Congress on Medicaid and CHIP,* which provided the foundation for a better understanding of the Medicaid and CHIP programs. It served as a starting point for building the analytic framework the Commission will use to assess access, evaluate payment policy, and determine key data needs in future work.

The Commission's authorizing language directs MACPAC to focus its June reports to the Congress on "issues affecting Medicaid and CHIP, including the implications of changes in health care delivery in the United States and in the market for health care services on such programs." Medicaid finances health care and related services for about 67 million individuals, including more than 30 million low-income children, more than 10 million persons with disabilities, and 6 million low-income seniors with Medicare. Of these 67 million people, there are approximately 49 million low-income individuals enrolled in some form of Medicaid managed care. Understanding Medicaid managed care arrangements is essential to determining how the program fits into U.S. health care.

The Commission's June 2011 Report to the Congress is comprised of two major sections: a baseline description of managed care in Medicaid, and Medicaid and CHIP Program Statistics (MACStats), a standing supplement in MACPAC Reports that provides national and state-specific data on enrollees, spending, and program features.

The first section of the Report provides a comprehensive resource on what is known about the use of managed care in Medicaid today, both nationally and at the state level. The majority of states use managed care, and these arrangements are likely to become even more prevalent over the coming years. However, Medicaid managed care programs vary considerably among states, as well as within states, across different populations, and geographic locations. This Report describes the enrollees in Medicaid managed care, including children and families, enrollees with disabilities, and those who are dually eligible for Medicaid and Medicare. The current status of enrollment, payment, access, and quality measurement and improvement is examined, as well as the consistency, availability, and timeliness of data needed to adequately evaluate managed care programs and ensure program accountability.

The Commission's June 2011 edition of MACStats presents data on all enrollee groups but highlights enrollment, service use, spending, and characteristics of individuals with disabilities. We focus on these high cost, high need enrollees because they account for a substantial portion of the program's spending, although they are a small share of enrollment. This is a key issue for policymakers as they consider options for controlling spending and improving care management for the complex needs of this population.

Moving forward, the Commission plans to examine policies to encourage high quality, efficient care for all enrollees in managed care and in traditional fee for service, especially for those who have complex medical conditions. In addition, the Commission is undertaking research and independent data analysis on access to develop an early-warning system as described in our statutory charge. In this effort, we will work to identify provider shortage areas and other factors that may affect access to care for those enrolled in Medicaid and CHIP.

The Commission provides non-partisan, data-driven advice to the Congress about how Medicaid and CHIP can work more effectively. We hope that this Report and the work of the Commission will serve to inform and assist the Congress in its deliberations.

Sincerely,

Diane Rowland

Diane Rowland, ScD
Chair

Enclosure

Acknowledgements

The Commission would like to thank the many people who contributed to this June 2011 *Report to the Congress: The Evolution of Managed Care in Medicaid.*

State officials offered valuable insight and assistance. In particular, we would like to thank Andrew Allison, Nancy Atkins, Roberta Bradford, Toby Douglas, Mike Fogarty, Stephen Fitton, Darin Gordon, Jason Helgerson, and Susan Moran.

Thank you to the staff of the Department of Health and Human Services particularly the Centers for Medicare & Medicaid Services for their contributions, including Dan Aibel, Henry Claypool, Mindy Cohen, Camille Dobson, Pamela Doty, John Drabek, Gavin Kennedy, John Klemm, Don Kosin, and Chris Truffer.

This Report also benefited from the contributions of many experts with experience in managed care and Medicaid on both the federal and state level, including Christine Aguiar, Joesph Antos, Andrew Bindman, Gretchen Brown, Robin Cohen, Christine Coyer, Jennifer Edwards, Mike Fiore, Charlene Frizzera, Rachel Garfield, Marsha Gold, Catherine Hess, Jack Hoadley, Julie Hudman, Bruce Johnson, Neva Kaye, Genevieve Kenney, Jennifer Lee, Sharon Long, Alix Love, Andrea Maresca, Meg Murray, Michael Nardone, Jessica Nysenbaum, Richard Rimkunas, Candy Schaller, Vern Smith, Karen Stockley, Sarah Thomas, Julie Topoleski, Sid Trieger, Patricia Votava, Howard Weiss, and Carlos Zarabozo.

Finally, the Commission would also like to thank Kerri Cornejo, Imelda Demus, Yajaira Gijon, Elizabeth Hargrave, Wilhelmine Miller, and their colleagues at NORC at the University of Chicago for their assistance in editing and producing this Report.

Table of Contents

List of Tables

List of Figures

List of Boxes

Report Summary

Medicaid is a source of health care coverage for 67 million low-income people, over a fifth of the U.S. population.[1] Medicaid finances health care and related services for more than 30 million low-income children, more than 10 million persons with disabilities, and 6 million low-income seniors with Medicare. Approximately 49 million Medicaid enrollees receive care through some form of Medicaid managed care. Understanding the different Medicaid managed care arrangements and the interactions between states, plans, providers, enrollees, and the federal government is important to understanding how the Medicaid program—which accounts for approximately 15 percent of U.S. health care spending—fits into the larger health care delivery system.

MACPAC's June 2011 *Report to the Congress: The Evolution of Managed Care in Medicaid* establishes a baseline of what is known about the use of managed care in Medicaid today. This Report builds upon the foundational information on Medicaid and CHIP and the Commission's analytic framework on access and payment presented in its March 2011 *Report to the Congress on Medicaid and CHIP*.

The June 2011 *Report to the Congress: The Evolution of Managed Care in Medicaid* consists of two parts. First, the Commission presents a baseline description of managed care in Medicaid. This part of the Report is divided into seven policy areas:

- Section A: Context and Overview of Medicaid Managed Care
- Section B: Populations and Enrollment in Medicaid Managed Care
- Section C: Managed Care Plans
- Section D: Payment Policy in Medicaid Managed Care
- Section E: Access and Quality in Managed Care
- Section F: Program Accountability, Integrity, and Data
- Section G: Issues Facing Medicaid and CHIP Managed Care

Second, in MACStats—the Medicaid and CHIP program statistics supplement in the gray-banded portion of the Report—the Commission presents state-level information on Medicaid populations. This edition of MACStats presents data on all enrollee groups but highlights enrollment, service use, spending, and characteristics of individuals with disabilities in part because they are high cost, high need enrollees but also because they account for a substantial share of the program's spending, but a small portion of enrollment. This is a key issue for policymakers as they consider options for controlling

[1] U.S. territories excluded.

spending and improving care management for the complex needs of these populations.

The MACStats portion of the Report is divided into four sections:

▷ Section 1: Trends in Medicaid Enrollment and Spending

▷ Section 2: Medicaid and CHIP Populations

▷ Section 3: Medicaid Managed Care

▷ Section 4: Technical Guide to the June 2011 MACStats

The Evolution of Medicaid Managed Care

Medicaid managed care arrangements differ from those in the private sector and in Medicare in part due to differences in the populations served. Enrollment of low-income populations (e.g., at or below 133 percent of the federal poverty level or $24,645 a year for a family of three) with limited resources and often complex health needs affects Medicaid managed care program design. The role of provider networks, the use of cost sharing as a tool for managing utilization, the enrollment process, and the types of organizations sponsoring managed care plans differ from the private sector and Medicare managed care plans. These distinct differences can affect whether and how states use managed care in Medicaid to deliver quality care.

The term "managed care" may refer to several different arrangements for delivering and financing health care services. About 71 percent of all Medicaid enrollees receive care in a managed care arrangement, including comprehensive risk-based plans, primary care case management (PCCM) programs, and limited-benefit plans.[2] The design, operation, covered populations, and covered

services of Medicaid managed care vary from state to state. Some states rely on PCCMs or limited-benefit plans rather than comprehensive risk-based plans because of their geography, provider base, populations or preferences.

Most state Medicaid managed care programs focus primarily on low-income children and families, although some use managed care arrangements for populations with more extensive medical needs, such as Medicaid enrollees with disabilities. States that have implemented managed care programs are likely to move in this direction in the near future as they seek to control costs and better coordinate care for high need, high cost populations, particularly as they continue to struggle with their budgets.

MACPAC's June 2011 *Report to the Congress: The Evolution of Managed Care in Medicaid* provides a baseline examination of Medicaid managed care, including information on enrolled populations, managed care plan arrangements, payment policy, access and quality, program accountability, program integrity, and data. The Report contains the Commission's initial review of the current state of Medicaid managed care and its role in Medicaid, both nationally and at the state level. The Report highlights:

Trends in Enrollment (See MACStats Tables 9 and 11). Comprehensive risk-based managed care enrollment in Medicaid is growing nationwide, and the population covered is expanding to enrollees with disabilities.

▷ Medicaid enrollment in comprehensive risk-based programs has increased to 47 percent of enrollees in 2009, up from 15 percent in 1995.

▷ Low-income children and non-disabled adults under age 65 were most likely to be enrolled

---

[2] MACPAC's estimate of national managed care enrollment (71 percent) differs from that reported by CMS (72 percent) due to the exclusion of the territories.

in comprehensive risk-based managed care (60 percent and 44 percent respectively) in FY 2008 than other groups.

- Individuals with disabilities were enrolled in comprehensive risk-based programs in 39 states and the District of Columbia in FY 2008; 28 percent of all Medicaid enrollees with disabilities are enrolled in comprehensive risk-based managed care. However, the percentage of this group's enrollment in comprehensive risk-based managed care varies significantly by state—from less than 1 percent to over 90 percent.

- Low-income seniors, mostly with primary coverage through Medicare, were the least likely to be enrolled in comprehensive risk-based managed care: 11 percent of all Medicaid enrollees age 65 and older were enrolled in comprehensive risk-based managed care programs in FY 2008.

Managed Care Arrangements (See MACStats Tables 9 and 10). States choose managed care arrangements and/or fee for service (FFS) depending on their unique populations, provider base, benefits, geography, and state goals.

- Thirty-four states and the District of Columbia had comprehensive risk-based Medicaid managed care programs in 2009, with 21 states and the District of Columbia enrolling more than half of their total Medicaid population in such programs.[3] Many of the 16 states without comprehensive risk-based plans are largely rural.

- Thirty states used PCCM programs to coordinate care in FFS and 34 states and the District of Columbia used limited-benefit plans to provide selected services (such as behavioral health and oral health) in managed care and FFS settings.

- Thirty-seven states and the District of Columbia used a combination of two or more managed care arrangements and 13 states used all three managed care approaches in their Medicaid programs.[4]

- Using the CMS definition, 71 percent of Medicaid enrollees in 2009 were enrolled in some form of managed care arrangement in 48 states and the District of Columbia. Most Medicaid enrollees still receive at least some services through FFS arrangements.

Payment Policy. There is considerable variation in the way states pay managed care plans.

- States with comprehensive risk-based managed care generally use forms of administered pricing or competitive bidding to establish payment rates for plans. Rates are required to be actuarially sound.

- States use different methods of adjusting payments to reflect the health and demographic characteristics of enrollees. More analysis is needed on risk adjustment models for complex, low-income populations.

- For some states, moving populations into managed care has implications for certain FFS supplemental payments.

---

[3] Seven additional states have Program for All-Inclusive Care for the Elderly (PACE) programs but no other comprehensive risk-based managed care.

[4] Excludes PACE programs.

Access, Quality, and Program Accountability.
Monitoring access to care, quality, and program integrity effectively in Medicaid managed care requires current, reliable data and sound data analysis.

▷ The consistency, availability, and timeliness of the data submitted by managed care plans to states and subsequently from states to CMS vary considerably, creating challenges for analyzing and monitoring managed care programs and policies at the national level and limiting the ability to create baseline data and compare states.

▷ Multistate data and analyses on managed care arrangements would better enable monitoring of program integrity, appropriate utilization of health care services, and access to care.

Highlights of each managed care section of the report include:

Section A: Context and Overview of Medicaid Managed Care

Many states have pursued managed care as a tool to provide greater control and predictability over Medicaid spending, better coordinate care for enrollees, and establish provider networks for low-income enrollees. However, FFS continues to be an important component of Medicaid program design and spending.

▷ Forty-eight states and the District of Columbia have some form of managed care for all or part of their Medicaid program.

▷ Over 49 million Medicaid enrollees (71 percent of total Medicaid enrollees) were enrolled in some form of managed care in 2009.

▷ Managed care accounts for 40 percent of all Medicaid spending on children and 21 percent of total Medicaid spending.

Managed care arrangements in Medicaid vary from those in the private sector and in Medicare due to differences in populations served, program design, and history. In particular, there are distinct differences in the role of provider networks, the use of cost sharing as a tool for managing utilization, the enrollment process, and the types of organizations sponsoring managed care plans in different markets. These differences affect whether and how states use managed care to deliver quality care.

Federal parameters guiding state use of managed care in Medicaid have evolved over time, shaping how states design their managed care delivery systems, and whom they enroll. As states and the federal government look for ways to curb and control Medicaid spending growth, managed care is being examined as a potential vehicle for improving care and generating savings.

Section B: Populations and Enrollment in Medicaid Managed Care

Medicaid enrollees are a diverse population and each Medicaid eligibility group (i.e., low-income children, adults, individuals with disabilities, seniors) varies considerably in their health characteristics, service use, and spending, creating different opportunities and challenges for enrollment in managed care.

When large expansions of Medicaid enrollment into managed care began in the mid-1990's the focus was on children and families. Historically, enrollees with disabilities and enrollees age 65 and older were generally excluded or exempted from enrollment in managed care and received their Medicaid benefits through either FFS or small demonstrations or voluntary programs that attracted few enrollees. Because these two populations combined account for only 25 percent of Medicaid enrollees, states can obtain high managed care enrollment by enrolling only children and families. However, there is growing interest among states to extend managed care to enrollees with disabilities and enrollees age 65 and older. Both groups tend to have more complex health care needs and higher costs than children and families. In addition, many seniors and some Medicaid enrollees with disabilities also have Medicare which may complicate coordination and state choices.

This section of the Report describes the populations who are enrolled in managed care and their share of Medicaid spending. It also examines the Medicaid managed care enrollment process and related issues such as enrollee outreach and education, plan choice, and auto-assignment. State rationales for pursuing managed care for enrollees with disabilities and dual eligible populations (individuals enrolled in both Medicare and Medicaid) and the issues regarding enrolling high need, high cost populations into managed care are also described.

Section C: Managed Care Plans

Within Medicaid managed care, states use different types of arrangements to deliver services to enrollees including: comprehensive risk-based managed care, PCCM, and limited-benefit plans. These models differ in design, operation, and benefits covered. Measures of Medicaid managed care enrollment vary, depending on which models are included in total CMS enrollment numbers. In 2009, Medicaid managed care enrollment on average nationwide was:

▸ 71 percent of Medicaid enrollees when all three types of managed care are counted;

▸ 61 percent of Medicaid enrollees when only comprehensive risk-based plans or PCCM arrangements are counted; and

▸ 47 percent of Medicaid enrollees when only comprehensive risk-based plans are counted.

States are increasingly relying on comprehensive risk-based managed care; from 1995 to 2009 enrollment in comprehensive risk-based plans grew from 15 percent of Medicaid enrollees to 47 percent. However, many states with comprehensive risk-based plans also have PCCM programs within the state, particularly in rural areas where attracting and retaining comprehensive risk-based plans or gaining provider support for managed care can be difficult. In 2009 over 30 states operated PCCM programs and eight states had more than 50 percent of their enrollment in PCCM arrangements.

This section of the Report highlights characteristics of and distinctions between various Medicaid managed care models and their use by states. It also discusses services that are commonly carved out of comprehensive risk-based plans.

Section D: Payment Policy in Medicaid Managed Care

Medicaid managed care payments vary in amount and complexity depending on the populations served, benefit packages provided, and whether the plans are at risk for the costs of services. This section primarily focuses on risk-based plans to which states typically make per member per month capitation payments. States use a variety of different approaches for setting payment rates for these risk-based plans, including risk adjustment and risk sharing methodologies.

State capitated rates are required to be actuarially sound, meaning they must be developed in accordance with generally accepted actuarial principles and practices; appropriate for the population and services; and certified by qualified actuaries. In setting rates, states must use applicable base utilization and cost data and account for enrollee characteristics. Many states have begun to use risk adjustment, using a variety of different approaches to adjust rates based on enrollee health status. This allows rates to better reflect the mix of enrollees in each plan and to better predict expenditures.

Additionally, some states may share risk with Medicaid managed care plans through risk corridors or stop-loss arrangements that mitigate a plan's financial loss when plan expenses exceed capitated payment rates. High cost enrollees may be excluded from managed care plans as well to help lower the risk borne by plans.

This section of the Report provides an overview of the federal statutes and regulations that govern Medicaid payment to managed care plans; some of the state approaches to determining managed care payment rates; and methods used by states to mitigate plan risk, namely risk adjustment and risk sharing.

Section E: Access and Quality in Managed Care

Managed care arrangements including comprehensive risk-based plans and PCCM programs link enrollees with a primary care provider and case management, and in doing so may offer opportunities for improved continuity and care coordination. In addition, managed care programs are intended to emphasize care management. Poorly designed or implemented Medicaid managed care systems can create issues for states that may lead to poor enrollee health outcomes.

Standards, reporting, and enforcement of managed care contract requirements vary considerably across states, and there are no uniform sets of measures or data sources used by states that could provide comparability of data for assessing access and quality nationally. The existing data and analyses for

addressing access are limited and dated. The ability to synthesize research across states is constrained since individual studies typically focus on only one or a few states and vary in comprehensiveness, measurement use, and research quality.

In this section of the Report, the Commission reviews how access and quality are evaluated and monitored in Medicaid managed care. This section also describes quality measurement and improvement activities most commonly used by states.

Section F: Program Accountability, Integrity, and Data

Appropriate payment and access to quality care in Medicaid managed care programs and preventing fraud, waste, and abuse is a responsibility of both the federal government and the states. CMS sets broad operational and administrative requirements related to payment rates, provider availability in plan networks, provision of health care services, and quality of care for Medicaid enrollees in managed care. Within these parameters, states have flexibility in how they design and administer their programs and monitor participating managed care plans. Monitoring the effectiveness of managed care in Medicaid requires a considerable amount of data exchange among the plans, the states, and the federal government.

Effective methods for monitoring Medicaid managed care program integrity (PI) efforts at the state and plan level depends on state systems and their ability to identify problems. Data reported by managed care plans and states provide important information for states and the federal government for addressing key policy and accountability questions. Data can be used to track trends and make projections on spending, service use, and the quality and appropriateness of care. While managed care plans submit certain data to states and states report certain data to CMS, the consistency, availability, and timeliness of the data submitted vary considerably among states. This creates challenges for analyzing and monitoring managed care programs and policies across the country and limits the ability to compare states.

This section of the Report examines state and federal administration and oversight of Medicaid managed care programs and highlights PI requirements at the state and federal level to ensure proper payment for appropriate, high quality care in both FFS and managed care. This section also discusses data for policy development and program accountability and some of the challenges and limitations in current data collection for Medicaid managed care. Lastly, this section contains two annexes that outline (1) key federal authorities allowing Medicaid managed care and (2) comprehensive risk-based contract requirements.

Section G: Issues Facing Medicaid and CHIP Managed Care

As a way to improve care management and care coordination, secure provider networks for beneficiaries, lower spending or make it more predictable, and improve program accountability, states have pursued managed care strategies. All of these goals will continue to be important as states work to improve the health of Medicaid enrollees, both in managed care and FFS, while addressing budget constraints. However, state strategies are likely to differ based on factors such as population characteristics, population density, provider availability, plan participation, state goals, and existing managed care arrangements in each state.

In this section of the Report, the Commission identifies some of the issues state Medicaid programs will encounter as they consider expanding existing or developing new managed care programs. The topics addressed in this Report will continue to be salient: enrollment, plan participation and benefit design, payment, access to care and care quality, and data for program accountability and integrity. Building on the baseline data in this Report, the Commission will seek to provide a better understanding of these issues as the basis for future work on how health care delivery and financing can work more effectively for Medicaid and CHIP enrollees.

MACStats: Medicaid and CHIP Program Statistics

MACStats is a standing section in all MACPAC reports to the Congress. It was created because data and information on the Medicaid and CHIP programs can often be difficult to find and are spread out across a variety of sources. The June 2011 edition of MACStats illustrates trends in Medicaid enrollment and spending, as well as current health and other characteristics, service use, and spending among Medicaid and CHIP populations. It also supplements the Report's Medicaid managed care sections with state-level data on Medicaid managed care plans, enrollment, and spending.

In addition to state-level data by eligibility group, data highlighting users of long-term services and supports (LTSS) and other enrollee subgroups such as children with special health care needs are presented. These data illustrate how Medicaid populations differ in terms of their characteristics, service use, and spending.

The Evolution of Managed Care in Medicaid

SECTION

Context and Overview of Medicaid Managed Care

Medicaid is a source of health care coverage for 67 million people, over a fifth of the U.S. population. Approximately 49 million Medicaid enrollees receive care through some form of managed care.

Managed care may encompass many different arrangements for financing or delivering health care. As described later in this section, managed care arrangements range from comprehensive risk-based plans and primary care case management (PCCM) programs in Medicaid to preferred provider organizations (PPOs) and traditional health maintenance organizations (HMOs) in employer-sponsored plans. In one form or another, these health plan arrangements have grown to be the dominant approach to delivering and financing health care services in the United States. However, fee for service (FFS) continues to be an important component of Medicaid program design and spending.

A few states have been using managed care in Medicaid since the early years of the program, but enrollment has expanded more rapidly in the last 15 years. In 2009, 47 percent of all Medicaid enrollees were enrolled in comprehensive risk-based managed care plans, up from 15 percent in 1995 (CMS 1996, CMS 2010). These comprehensive risk-based plans are responsible for providing a varying but relatively inclusive set of Medicaid benefits for a fixed per member per month amount.[1]

Within Medicaid, the term "managed care" has come to include a broader array of arrangements beyond comprehensive risk-based plans. About 15 percent of Medicaid enrollees are in PCCM programs that build on FFS arrangements using

---

[1] In this Report, the term "comprehensive risk-based plans" refers to what federal Medicaid regulations generally call a managed care organization, which covers comprehensive services (42 CFR 438.2). In the federal Medicaid regulations, comprehensive services are defined as (a) inpatient hospital services and at least one of the following nine services, or (b) any three of the following nine services: (1) outpatient hospital services; (2) rural health clinic services; (3) federally qualified health center (FQHC) services; (4) other laboratory and X-ray services; (5) nursing facility (NF) services; (6) early and periodic screening, diagnostic, and treatment (EPSDT) services; (7) family planning services; (8) physician services; and (9) home health services.

care coordination and care management.[2] To complement FFS and managed care arrangements, under which enrollees may receive most of their benefits, many states use limited-benefit plans (i.e., prepaid ambulatory health plans (PAHPs) and prepaid inpatient health plans (PIHPs)) to provide a particular service such as behavioral health, transportation, or oral health.

Although most Medicaid managed care programs primarily enroll low-income[3] children and their parents, some states use managed care arrangements for populations with more extensive medical needs, including persons with disabilities. As they seek to control costs and better coordinate care for these enrollees, states may rely more on managed care in the near future. In addition, changes in Medicaid eligibility rules in 2014 will potentially bring new populations and new issues for the use of managed care in Medicaid.

Identifying payment, access, quality, and other strategies for improving managed care is important for current Medicaid and State Children's Health Insurance Program (CHIP) populations and for future enrollees in these programs. Critical to the success of these improvement strategies is the availability of data. While states may have the data they need to operate their programs, insufficient information is available at the national level to conduct data-based analyses across states of what works and what could be improved.

Comprehensive risk-based managed care programs are the primary focus of this Report. However, we also provide information on the PCCM programs states use as an alternative when comprehensive risk-based managed care is less feasible or desirable, such as for certain geographic areas or

populations. Limited-benefit plans are considered mainly from the perspective of which benefits are carved out of the comprehensive risk-based managed care plan benefit package.

This Report establishes baseline information about the use of managed care in Medicaid today, including data on populations and enrollment, types of Medicaid managed care plans, payment policy, access and quality issues, and program accountability. A program statistics supplement, MACStats, is also included in the Report and provides state-level data on Medicaid managed care including data on plans as well as enrollment and spending by eligibility group. In addition, MACStats provides information on the historical growth in Medicaid spending as well as the demographic and health characteristics of individuals enrolled in Medicaid and CHIP, as compared to other sources of coverage and among subgroups within the Medicaid and CHIP populations.

A Focus on Managed Care in Medicaid

The Commission's authorizing language directs the Commission to focus its June report to the Congress on "issues affecting Medicaid and CHIP, including the implications of changes in health care delivery in the United States and in the market for health care services on such programs." Understanding managed care's use in Medicaid and CHIP is essential to understanding how these two programs—which together account for approximately 15 percent of U.S. health care spending—fit into the larger health care delivery system (MACPAC 2011).

---

[2] See MACStats Table 9.

[3] Based on 2010 estimates from the National Health Interview Survey, 48 percent of Medicaid enrollees had incomes below 100 percent of poverty; 32 percent had incomes between 100 and 199 percent of poverty; and 20 percent had incomes above 200 percent of poverty (March 2011 MACStats Table 18). One hundred percent of poverty using Census' poverty threshold was $17,098 for a family of three.

States and the federal government have pursued Medicaid managed care for a number of reasons. When designed and implemented well, effective managed care programs may:

▷ promote care management and care coordination;

▷ provide greater control and predictability over state spending; and

▷ improve program accountability for performance, access, and quality.

However, for some states, FFS may still provide advantages for certain populations and certain geographic areas.

Despite the widespread use of Medicaid managed care, most research is dated or narrowly focused on single states. It is essential to develop a new generation of in-depth research that addresses how states are meeting their goals for Medicaid managed care and identifies how programs can be updated and strengthened as states move to enroll more individuals.

The Commission's work will provide a foundation needed to examine the trends, opportunities, and challenges in fundamental policy areas including the impact of payment policy, access to care, and appropriate utilization of services. Over time, our analyses will aim to identify potential ways for the federal government and states to improve managed care payment, enrollment processes, quality improvement activities, and program integrity.

BOX A-1. Key Facts on Managed Care in Medicaid

Enrollees
(Table B-1)

▷ Percent of Medicaid managed care enrollees, by eligibility status, who are in any form of managed care (including comprehensive risk-based, PCCM, or limited-benefit arrangements):

  ▫ Non-disabled children: 60%

  ▫ Non-disabled adults under age 65: 22%

  ▫ Persons with disabilities: 14%

  ▫ Individuals age 65 and over: 4%

Enrollment
(Table 9 in MACStats)

▷ Number of Medicaid enrollees in any form of managed care: 49 million (71%)

▷ Number of Medicaid enrollees in comprehensive risk-based managed care: 23 million (47%)

  ▫ States with highest percent of Medicaid enrollees in comprehensive risk-based managed care: Hawaii (97%), Tennessee (94%), and Arizona (90%)

Spending
(Table B-2)

▷ Share of Medicaid benefit spending for any form of managed care: 21%

▷ Share of Medicaid benefit spending for comprehensive risk-based managed care: 18%

States
(Table 9 in MACStats
and CMS 2010)

▷ Number of state Medicaid programs with:

  ▫ Comprehensive risk-based managed care plans: 34 states and DC

  ▫ PCCM programs: 30 states

  ▫ Limited-benefit plans: 34 states and DC

  ▫ No managed care: 2 states (Alaska and Wyoming)

Notes: See Section 4 of MACStats for further explanation of methodology and differences in data sources. Data are from 2009 except spending and enrollee data, which are from FY 2008.

TABLE A-1. Percentage of Medicaid Enrollees in Managed Care by Type of Arrangement, FY 2008

	Children	Adults	Disabled	Aged
Any managed care	84.6%	57.1%	58.4%	32.9%
Comprehensive risk-based plans	60.0	43.8	27.9	10.9
Primary care case management (PCCM)	19.0	8.9	12.6	2.1
Limited-benefit plans	36.6	23.6	37.0	25.2

Notes: Managed care types do not sum to total because individuals are counted in every category for which a payment was made on their behalf during the year. Excludes the territories and Medicaid-expansion CHIP enrollees. Children and non-aged adults who qualify for Medicaid on the basis of a disability are included in the disabled category. Enrollees are counted as participating in managed care if at least one managed care payment was made on their behalf during the fiscal year; this method underestimates participation somewhat because it misses enrollees who entered managed care late in the year but for whom a payment was not made until the following fiscal year. See Section 4 and Tables 11 and 12 in MACStats for more information on how MSIS data used for this table differ from Medicaid Managed Care Enrollment Report data used throughout this Report.

Source: MACPAC analysis of Medicaid Statistical Information System (MSIS) annual person summary (APS) data from CMS as of May 2011

As it continues to evolve, managed care in Medicaid will continue to be dependent on effective working relationships between federal and state governments, states and managed care plans, and managed care plans and participating providers. This Report touches on all of these relationships and identifies the roles and responsibilities of each entity.

Medicaid and Managed Care

Three different types of arrangements in Medicaid are often referred to as managed care: comprehensive risk-based plans, PCCM programs and limited-benefit plans.

Comprehensive risk-based managed care plans are the most common type of managed care arrangements in Medicaid. States typically use a HMO model in which enrollees must use a network of providers. States pay plans on a capitated basis—a set amount per member per month that covers all benefits and services under the plan contract—but may mitigate some of the plans' risk through risk corridors or other

arrangements designed to limit plan losses. In 2009, 23 million Medicaid enrollees (47 percent of all enrollees) were in comprehensive risk-based plans (MACStats Table 9).

PCCM programs typically assure that enrollees have a primary care provider (PCP) who receives a small monthly per capita payment to coordinate each enrollee's care. All services are still paid on a FFS basis. In 2009, 7.3 million Medicaid enrollees (15 percent of all enrollees) were in PCCM programs (MACStats Table 9).

Limited-benefit plans include a diverse assortment of plans that typically cover only a single type of benefit. Generally paid on a capitated basis, these arrangements can be used in conjunction with either of the other two types of managed care programs or with FFS Medicaid. Among Medicaid enrollees in limited-benefit plans, 4.3 million were in plans covering inpatient mental health services and 3.1 million were in plans with combined inpatient mental health and substance abuse benefits; 6.1 million enrollees were in plans that provided transportation services only. Dental limited-benefit plans accounted for 1.2 million enrollees in five states (CMS 2010).

States differ considerably in the populations they enroll in managed care, the roles and responsibilities they assign to managed care plans, the level of oversight and management they retain at the state level, and the maturity of their programs. For example, in 2009, four states had at least three-fourths of their Medicaid enrollees in comprehensive risk-based managed care plans, while 13 other states with comprehensive risk-based managed care used that arrangement for less than half of their enrollees (MACStats Table 9). Some states mandate managed care enrollment of certain enrollees while others maintain only voluntary programs that allow enrollees to choose between enrolling in managed care or remaining in FFS. Furthermore, different geographic regions of a state may be treated differently; even in states that rely heavily on managed care, some geographic regions may not be included, especially in rural areas.

States typically have implemented managed care on a population-by-population basis. Low-income children and their parents were the first

population that states began enrolling in managed care on a regular basis, and they are by far the most commonly enrolled population in all three types of managed care arrangements (Table A-1). Sixty percent of all children in Medicaid are enrolled in a comprehensive risk-based plan. Non-disabled adults under age 65—typically parents of Medicaid-eligible children—are the next most likely to be enrolled in comprehensive risk-based managed care (44 percent). Only 28 percent of enrollees with disabilities and 11 percent of enrollees age 65 and older are in comprehensive risk-based managed care. These two groups are more likely to be in a limited-benefit plan (such as those for behavioral health) than any other arrangement (Table A-1).

CHIP and Managed Care

With the creation of CHIP in 1997, states were given the option to administer their CHIP programs through Medicaid (called a Medicaid-expansion program), as a separate, stand-alone program, or by using a combination of the two programs (see March 2011 Report for additional details).

TABLE A-2. Child CHIP Enrollment in Managed Care Plans, FY 2010

	Medicaid-expansion CHIP		Separate CHIP		Total	
Comprehensive risk-based	1,241,441	57%	4,503,711	81%	5,745,152	75%
Fee for service (FFS)	450,253	21	778,354	14	1,228,607	16
Primary care case management (PCCM)	474,256	22	257,708	5	731,964	9
Total	2,165,950	100%	5,539,773	100%	7,705,723	100%

Note: In the CHIP Statistical Enrollment Data System (SEDS), information is not obtained on limited-benefit plans.
Source: MACPAC analysis (February 2011) of SEDS, as reported by states, based on their definitions

Comprehensive risk-based plans are prominent in both separate CHIP programs and Medicaid-expansion CHIP programs. In 2010 three out of four CHIP enrollees were in such plans, including 81 percent of children in separate CHIP programs (Table A-2). Medicaid-expansion CHIP programs typically use the same plans as a state's overall Medicaid program and are more likely than stand-alone CHIP programs to use PCCM or FFS arrangements.

Relatively little research compares managed care in separate CHIP programs to Medicaid-expansion CHIP programs. In CHIP, managed care is less than one-fifth the size of the Medicaid managed care market. However, a 2007 study found that CHIP managed care enrollees were served by a slightly larger percentage of commercial plans: 35 percent of all commercial plans participated in CHIP compared to 29 percent in Medicaid (Barrett and Felt-Lisk 2008). A 2001 study comparing six states with stand-alone programs to five states with Medicaid-expansion CHIP programs found that the plans participating in both Medicaid and CHIP overlapped substantially (Gold et al. 2003).

Beyond these general statistics and limited studies, little information is currently available on the managed care arrangements states use in their stand-alone CHIP programs. Additional data are helpful to better understand these CHIP programs, their enrollment processes, the plans that participate and payment policies. Further, little is known about how CHIP stand-alone programs perform compared to Medicaid. The Commission intends to focus more on managed care in CHIP as part of our future work.

Medicaid Managed Care in the Context of U.S. Health Care

Managed care arrangements in Medicaid, in the private sector and in Medicare differ in several ways. These differences stem in large part from the differences in the populations served, how the programs are designed, statutory requirements for the programs, and their history. Key differences include:

- the role of provider networks;
- the role of cost sharing as a tool for managing utilization; and
- the process for enrolling in a managed care plan and the plan choices available at enrollment.

This section provides further background on how design features of managed care in Medicaid are similar to and different from those most commonly used in the private sector and Medicare markets.

The role of provider networks. Historically, managed care plans have generally sought to control costs by establishing a network of providers to provide health services to plan members. Contracts between the plan and participating providers typically stipulate the negotiated payment amount and how those payments will be administered. Providers may accept payments lower than their usual rates in exchange for having access to the plan's enrollees.

In 2010, most individuals in employer-sponsored plans were enrolled in PPOs (58 percent). PPOs encourage the use of network providers, but often cover services from non-network providers if enrollees pay an extra charge. Persons with employer-sponsored insurance were also enrolled in HMOs (19 percent), high deductible health plans with a savings option (13 percent), and point-of-service plans (8 percent) (KFF and HRET 2010).

Most Medicare enrollees have FFS coverage; in 2011 about one-fourth of beneficiaries are enrolled in Medicare Advantage (MA) managed care plans. Within MA, HMOs are the most common plan type, covering about 64 percent of enrollees in MA. PPOs account for about 20 percent of MA enrollment. Approximately 9 percent of MA enrollees are individuals who are dually eligible for Medicaid and Medicare and enrolled in Special Needs Plans—usually HMOs—specifically designed to serve that population (MedPAC 2010).

Cost sharing as a management tool. Cost sharing is a tool managed care plans use to influence enrollee behavior, but it is less commonly used in Medicaid because of the low-income population the program serves. The PPO model emphasizes cost sharing as a tool for managing the use of services.

Cost sharing in traditional Medicare is generally set as a percentage of a fixed fee schedule once the applicable deductible is met. MA plans are allowed to vary cost sharing from that of traditional Medicare as long as the cost sharing remains actuarially equivalent to FFS Medicare. This allows plans such as PPOs to vary cost sharing to encourage the use of provider networks.

The ability to use cost sharing in Medicaid managed care is limited (March 2011 MACStats Table 13). In Medicaid, most cost sharing is restricted to nominal levels and deductibles are rarely used.[4] The nominal cost-sharing plans might be allowed to charge for out-of-network providers may not be enough to drive enrollee behavior. Thus Medicaid managed care plans create defined networks to ensure beneficiaries will use the providers with whom they have negotiated in-network payment rates.

Plan choice and the enrollment process.
For participants in employer-sponsored health insurance, selecting a health plan is typically overseen by the employer's benefits office. Only about 52 percent of covered employees work for a firm that offers more than one health plan type; a choice of plans is more common in large firms than small firms (KFF and HRET 2010). Where a choice of plan exists, employees commonly select a plan option during an annual open enrollment period where employees consider the available array of plans using information packages, health fairs, and other tools made available by the employer or their representative.

Similarly, Medicare holds an annual open enrollment period and offers various printed and online information resources for beneficiaries interested in choosing an MA plan. However, the default option is that beneficiaries will receive benefits (other than outpatient prescription drug benefits under Medicare Part D) through traditional FFS Medicare. Medicare beneficiaries are enrolled in FFS unless they actively choose a managed care plan.

In Medicaid, states are required to provide their enrollees with a choice of at least two plans if enrollment in managed care is mandatory (except in certain rural areas) (42 CFR 438.52). Compared to both employer-sponsored insurance and Medicare, Medicaid enrollees are far more likely to move frequently in and out of managed care plans, usually due to changes in income that affect their eligibility for Medicaid (Ku et al. 2009).

---

[4] The Deficit Reduction Act (P.L. 109-171) authorized states to implement, at state option, alternative premiums and cost sharing (e.g., for non-preferred prescription drugs) for certain populations whose incomes exceed specified levels.

BOX A-2.   Major Medicaid Managed Care Legislative Milestones and Key Provisions

1962   Public Welfare Amendments of 1962 (P.L. 87-543) establish Section 1115, which gives broad authority to the
Secretary to "waive compliance to any of the requirements" of a number of sections of the Social Security Act (the
Act) for any "experimental, pilot or demonstration" projects.

1965   Medicaid is enacted (P.L. 89-97) as Title XIX of the Act.

1973   Health Maintenance Organization Act of 1973 (HMO Act of 1973, P.L. 93-222) establishes requirements for health
maintenance organizations (HMOs).

1976   Health Maintenance Organization Amendments of 1976 (HMOA 1976, P.L. 94-460) mandate that no more than 50
percent of enrollees in plans participating in Medicaid could be comprised of Medicaid or Medicare beneficiaries,
known as the "50/50" rule.

   ▶ Requires entities seeking risk contracts under Medicaid to meet federal HMO requirements.

   ▶ Amends the definition of "HMO" in the Act to coordinate with HMO Act of 1973; also re-defines "basic health
services" as referring to mandatory Medicaid services.

   ▶ Prohibits payments to organizations providing inpatient hospital services or any other mandated Medicaid
services on a prepaid risk basis that are not qualified as an HMO.

1981   Omnibus Budget Reconciliation Act of 1981 (OBRA 1981, P.L. 97-35) establishes Section 1915(b) freedom-of-
choice waivers to allow states to pursue mandatory managed care enrollment of certain Medicaid populations.

   ▶ Replaces the "50/50" rule of HMOA 1976 with the "75/25" rule, which allows Medicaid participation by plans
with 75 percent Medicaid or Medicare enrollees.

   ▶ Requires Medicaid capitation payments to be actuarially sound.

1997   Balanced Budget Act of 1997 (BBA, P.L. 105-33) permits states to require most Medicaid beneficiaries to enroll
in managed care plans without obtaining a Section 1115 or 1915(b) waiver. This change shifts the role of Section
1115 waivers to broad program development and redesign.

   ▶ Eliminates the "75/25" rule which had required that 25 percent of a Medicaid plan's enrollment be privately
insured.

   ▶ Requires states to develop and implement a quality assessment and improvement strategy, specifically
assuring coverage of emergency services, creating a system to address complaints, demonstrating adequate
capacity and services, and meeting certain quality assurance standards.

   ▶ Calls for independent review of managed care organization performance.

2005   Deficit Reduction Act of 2005 (P.L.109-171) permits states to use "benchmark" coverage instead of the regular
Medicaid benefits package for certain populations; and gives states more flexibility to require cost sharing for
Medicaid enrolles.

2010   Patient Protection and Affordable Care Act (P.L. 111-148) extends the Medicaid Drug Rebate Program (established
by the Omnibus Budget Reconciliation Act of 1990, P.L. 101-508) to Medicaid managed care plans effective March
23, 2010.

The Evolution of Managed Care within Medicaid

Medicaid has evolved from an entirely FFS program to include managed care in an increasing role. Box A-2 presents some of the key legislative milestones in this evolution within the Medicaid program.

The first statutory authority used to implement managed care in Medicaid actually predated the program's 1965 passage. The Public Welfare Amendments of 1962 (P.L. 87-543) created Section 1115 of the Social Security Act, providing the federal government authority to grant waivers for broad, structural changes to federal aid programs operated by states on a demonstration basis. In Medicaid, this came to include waiving Medicaid enrollees' free choice of participating providers and permitting mandatory managed care enrollment.

Most states that enrolled Medicaid beneficiaries in managed care during the first decade of the program were seeking to achieve lower and more predictable costs (Gold and Mittler 2000). However, concerns were raised that plans did not provide needed care or took advantage of capitated payments by enrolling only people who rarely used care. California's Medicaid program first started contracting with comprehensive risk-based managed care plans (then called prepaid health plans) on a pilot basis in 1968 (GAO 1995). When the state rapidly expanded enrollment in these plans in the 1970s, controversies arose around questionable marketing practices, poor delivery systems, and plan financial stability (Freund and Hurley 1995). This may have slowed the implementation of Medicaid managed care in other states. The Health Maintenance Organization Amendments of 1976 (P.L. 94-460) followed these experiences and tightened certain rules for HMOs in Medicaid.

In 1981 the Congress enacted the Omnibus Reconciliation Act of 1981 (OBRA 1981, P.L. 97-35), adding another option for state-level experimentation. It added Section 1915(b) waivers to permit states to limit enrollees' choice of participating providers, another way of allowing states to implement mandatory managed care for their Medicaid populations. However, states were required to limit their waivers to a certain geographic area or certain populations. The legislation also included controls on programs created with waiver authority, to address some of the problems seen in the earliest Medicaid managed care programs. Table FA-1 in the Section F Annex of this Report summarizes key federal authorities allowing Medicaid managed care.

Using primarily Section 1915(b) waiver authority, by 1990 about 2.3 million Medicaid enrollees were enrolled in managed care (Freund and Hurley 1995). Still, by 1991, fewer than 1 in 10 Medicaid enrollees were in any form of managed care (Holahan et al. 1998).

In 1993 states began using Section 1115 research and demonstration authority (Section 1115 waivers) to implement programs that combined managed care and eligibility expansions (Rowland and Hanson 1996, Hurley and Somers 2007). These waivers allowed states to create statewide programs and waived the requirement that at least 25 percent of enrollees in participating plans be from outside the Medicaid and Medicare programs.

During this time period, as some states moved to implement statewide, broad-based managed care programs with ambitious deadlines, issues arose around the adequacy of provider networks, education and marketing practices, payment, data systems, and oversight. However, by 1997 the federal government had approved 14 Medicaid statewide waivers, all of them mandatorily enrolling some individuals in managed care, with a total enrollment of 8 million enrollees. Most states used comprehensive risk-based plans as their primary model of managed care (Smith and Moore 2008).

The Balanced Budget Act of 1997 (BBA, P.L. 105-33) included three changes with implications for Medicaid managed care. The first was the creation of CHIP. Children had already been a focus of managed care enrollment in Medicaid programs, and states continued to expand managed care for children enrolled in this new program.

Second, the BBA made it possible for states to implement mandatory enrollment in managed care programs through amendments to their state plans, rather than just through waivers (except for dual eligibles, American Indians, and children with special needs). In exchange, states were required to meet specific managed care program requirements that included standards of access and procedures for monitoring the quality and appropriateness of care. Lastly, the legislation allowed the creation of Medicaid-only plans and repealed the "75/25" rule from OBRA 1981 requiring plans to have a minimum share of private insurance enrollees.

Over the 12 years between 1997 and 2009, enrollment in Medicaid managed care increased from 8 million to 49 million, with 23 million in comprehensive risk-based plans (CMS 2010). In some states, interest continues to grow in expanding managed care to additional enrollees, especially high cost, high need populations.

The Future of Managed Care within Medicaid

The trend toward the use of managed care in Medicaid is likely to continue. The incentives for some states to expand their use of Medicaid managed care—both for managing costs and for improving coordination of care—are not changing and may well grow stronger as states continue to face serious budget pressures (NGA and NASBO 2011). In a recent survey, 20 states said they anticipated some expansion in Medicaid managed care either geographically or to additional subgroups of enrollees in FY 2011, with additional enrollment in both comprehensive risk-based plans and PCCM programs (Smith et al. 2010).

Historically, mandatory use of Medicaid managed care has focused mostly on low-income children and parents. While these two populations of Medicaid enrollees are generally less healthy than individuals in the same age range who are enrolled in private insurance, their health care costs are far lower and more predictable than the costs of Medicaid enrollees with disabilities and enrollees age 65 and older. This made them an attractive population for managed care enrollment.

As managed care oversight and payment systems have matured, more states have considered mandating enrollment of children with special health care needs and adults with disabilities or offering these enrollees more options for enrolling in managed care. Many states have also sought out better ways to coordinate care for dual eligibles, often under separate initiatives. Because these populations typically have high health care costs, states facing budget pressures are examining whether managed care arrangements might better manage health care spending for these populations (Bella et al. 2008).

Federal officials reviewing new managed care expansion requests from states will likely do so in the context of anticipated changes in Medicaid in 2014. In particular, the Patient Protection and Affordable Care Act (PPACA, P.L. 111-148) requires states to establish coverage for nonelderly parents, childless adults, and adults with disabilities with incomes up to 138 percent of poverty.[5] For most states, this represents an expansion of coverage for most, if not all, of these population groups. Among the newly eligible groups, parents and childless adults are likely to be a prime focus for managed care.

The introduction of state health insurance exchanges as required by current law may also have effects on Medicaid and CHIP with respect to enrollment and eligibility determination, and the introduction of new standards for minimum benefits for private plans. PPACA (§1413, §2101(e), and §2201) requires a streamlined eligibility and enrollment process across Medicaid, CHIP, and the health insurance exchange in each state, to ensure that applicants are screened for eligibility for all programs and referred for enrollment in the appropriate program without the need to go through multiple application procedures.

Other policy provisions in PPACA, together with ongoing state initiatives, may encourage use of managed care for persons with disabilities and dual eligibles. For example, PPACA created a new office in CMS for dual eligibles to examine the feasibility of more integration of services between Medicaid and Medicare. PPACA also calls for the creation of accountable care organizations (ACOs)— networks of hospitals, doctors, and other health professionals that agree to share responsibility for the care received by patients.

These statutory changes underscore the usefulness of developing reliable data and analyses on Medicaid managed care policies within the dynamic context of the U.S. health care system.

---

[5] For individuals whose eligibility is determined using modified adjusted gross income starting in 2014, the eligibility limit is 133 percent of the FPL, plus states will apply an income disregard equal to 5 percent of the FPL. This means that an individual whose total income equals 138 percent of the FPL will only have 133 percent of the FPL counted when his or her Medicaid eligibility is determined.

References

Barrett, A., and S. Felt-Lisk. 2008. *An overview of the managed care in the SCHIP program, 2007.* Draft report. Washington, DC: Mathematica Policy Research.

Bella, M. et al. 2008. *Purchasing strategies to improve care management for complex populations: A national scan of state purchasers.* Princeton, NJ: Center for Health Care Strategies. http://www.chcs.org/usr_doc/Purchasing_Strategies_to_Improve_Care_Manageme.pdf.

Centers for Medicare & Medicaid Services (CMS), Department of Health and Human Services. 2010. *2009 Medicaid managed care enrollment report. Summary statistics as of June 30, 2009.* https://www.cms.gov/MedicaidDataSourcesGenInfo/04_MdManCrEnrllRep.asp.

Centers for Medicare & Medicaid Services (CMS), Department of Health and Human Services. 1996. *1995 Medicaid Managed Care Enrollment Report, Summary Statistics as of June 30, 1995.* Washington, DC: HHS.

Freund, D., and R. Hurley. 1995. Medicaid managed care: Contribution to issues of health reform. *Annual Review of Public Health* 16: 473-495.

General Accounting Office (GAO). 1995. *Medicaid managed care: More competition and oversight would improve California's expansion plan,* No. GAO/HEHS-95-87. Washington, DC: GAO. http://www.gao.gov/archive/1995/he95087.pdf.

Gold, M., and J. Mittler. 2000. Second generation Medicaid managed care: Can it deliver? *Health Care Financing Review* 22, no. 2: 29-47.

Gold, M., J. Mittler, D. Draper, and D. Rousseau. 2003. Participation of plans and providers in Medicaid and SCHIP managed care. *Health Affairs* 22, no. 1: 230-240.

Holahan, J., S. Zuckerman, A. Evenans and S. Rangarajan. 1998. Medicaid managed care in thirteen states. *Health Affairs* 17, no. 3: 43-63.

Hurley, R., and S. Somers. 2007. Medicaid managed care. In *Essentials of managed health care,* edited by Peter R. Kongstvedt. Sudbury, MA: Jones & Bartlett Learning.

Kaiser Family Foundation (KFF) and Health Research and Educational Trust (HRET). 2010. *Employer health benefits: 2010 annual survey.* Menlo Park, CA and Chicago, IL: KFF and HRET. http://ehbs.kff.org.

Ku, L., P. MacTaggart, F. Pervez, and S. Rosenbaum. 2009. *Improving Medicaid's continuity of coverage and quality of care. Report to the Association for Community Affiliated Plans.* Washington, DC: George Washington University Department of Health Policy. http://www.ahcahp.org/Portals/0/ACAP%20Docs/Improving%20Medicaid%20Final%20070209.pdf.

Medicare Payment Advisory Commission (MedPAC). 2010. *A data book: Health care spending and the Medicare program.* Washington, DC: MedPAC. http://www.medpac.gov/documents/jun10databookentirereport.pdf.

Medicaid and CHIP Payment and Access Commission (MACPAC). 2011. *March 2011 Report to the Congress on Medicaid and CHIP.* Washington, DC: MACPAC. http://www.macpac.gov/reports.

National Governors Association (NGA) and the National Association of State Budget Officers (NASBO). 2011. *The Fiscal Survey of States.* Washington, DC: NGA. http://www.nga.org/files/pdf/fss106.pdf.

Rowland, D., and K. Hanson. 1996. Medicaid: Moving to managed care. *Health Affairs* 15, no. 3: 150-152. http://content.healthaffairs.org/content/15/3/150.full.pdf.

Smith, V., K. Gifford, E. Ellis, et al. 2010. *Hoping for economic recovery, preparing for health reform: A look at Medicaid spending, coverage and policy trends.* Washington, DC: Kaiser Family Foundation (KFF). http://www.kff.org/medicaid/upload/8105.pdf.

Smith, D., and J. Moore. 2008. *Medicaid politics and policy, 1965–2007.* New Brunswick, NJ: Transaction Publishers.

SECTION

Populations and Enrollment in Medicaid Managed Care

States have expanded their use of comprehensive risk-based managed care for Medicaid enrollees, but not to the same extent for all populations. When large expansions of Medicaid enrollment into managed care began in the mid-1990s, the focus was on low-income children and families. Historically, enrollees with disabilities as well as people age 65 and older were often excluded or exempted from enrollment in comprehensive risk-based managed care; they generally received Medicaid benefits that were paid on a fee-for-service (FFS) basis, sometimes augmented with a primary care case management (PCCM) program or limited-benefit plans for certain services. More recently, states have expressed growing interest in extending managed care to enrollees age 65 and older and enrollees with disabilities—25 percent of all Medicaid enrollees—who tend to have higher costs and more complex health care needs. However, these changes present challenges as well as opportunities to states.

Non-disabled children and adults under age 65 make up the largest share of comprehensive risk-based managed care enrollees (88 percent) and account for 66 percent of total spending for comprehensive risk-based managed care (Table B-1). By contrast, individuals with disabilities account for 10 percent of total enrollees in comprehensive risk-based plans and 27 percent of spending on comprehensive risk-based plans. Overall, individuals with disabilities and those age 65 and older report poorer health status, have higher rates of specific health conditions, and use more health services than children and younger adults without disabilities (MACStats Tables 3A-5C).

This section describes:

» the populations enrolled in Medicaid managed care plans;

» the share of program expenditures among the populations enrolled; and

» the opportunities and challenges of managed care for different populations.

Managed Care Enrollment and Spending

Medicaid provided health coverage for 67 million low-income individuals in FY 2010.[1] Forty-eight percent of Medicaid/CHIP enrollees have incomes below 100 percent of poverty—a much higher share than for the population covered by private insurance. Almost three-fourths of enrollees were non-disabled children and adults (33 million and 17 million, respectively), and the remaining Medicaid enrollees were 11 million individuals with disabilities (16 percent) and 6 million individuals age 65 and older (9 percent) (MACPAC 2011). These subpopulations of enrollees vary considerably in their health care needs, service use, and spending.

Overall enrollment in Medicaid managed care increased in the last decade, although this growth varied depending on the type of managed care arrangement and eligibility group. For example, the share of non-disabled adults under age 65 in comprehensive risk-based plans grew in the first half of the decade, while the share of other Medicaid enrollees in this form of managed care was relatively stable. There was moderate growth in the share of enrollees in comprehensive risk-based managed care in the second half of the decade for all eligibility groups. In limited-benefit plans, the share of non-disabled adults under age 65 has remained stable while enrollment of other groups has increased. The share of enrollees in PCCM programs fluctuated during this period, with marginal growth overall.[2]

Enrollment by Eligibility Group

Data reported by states to CMS (Tables A-1 and B-1) show that 85 percent of all children in Medicaid are enrolled in some type of managed care; children also make up the majority of the Medicaid managed care population (60 percent). Fifty-seven percent of non-disabled adults under age 65 are enrolled in some form of managed care, making up 22 percent of the Medicaid managed care population. Persons with disabilities and those 65 and older are less likely to be enrolled in Medicaid managed care and therefore make up a much smaller share of Medicaid managed care enrollment (14 and 4 percent, respectively). Compared to child and adult enrollees, aged and disabled enrollees make up a smaller share of those in comprehensive risk-based plans (which is the main focus of this Report) and a larger share of those in limited-benefit plans (which generally cover services such as behavioral health and transportation). For more detail on the different types of Medicaid managed care arrangements, see Section C of this Report.

Spending by Eligibility Group

Total Medicaid spending varies across the different Medicaid subpopulations. Of $338.6 billion in total Medicaid benefit spending in FY 2008, 21 percent was for managed care (Table B-2). The largest share was for comprehensive risk-based plans, which accounted for 18 percent of all Medicaid benefit spending by states.[3] (See MACStats Table 12 for these data by state.) PCCM programs accounted for less than 1 percent of spending because most services provided to enrollees in PCCM programs are paid on a FFS basis; the only amounts tracked as managed care payments are the

---

[1] U.S. territories are excluded.

[2] MACPAC analysis of FY 2002–FY 2008 Medicaid Statistical Information System (MSIS) state summary data from CMS as of April 2011.

[3] States may also make FFS payments on behalf of individuals enrolled in these plans if they carve out certain services from the managed care plan contract. For more on this practice, see Section C of this Report.

TABLE B-1. Distribution of Managed Care Enrollees and Managed Care Spending by Eligibility Group, FY 2008

Basis of Eligibility	Any Managed Care		Comprehensive Risk-based Plans		Primary Care Case Management		Limited-benefit Plans	
	Enrollees	Spending	Enrollees	Spending	Enrollees	Spending	Enrollees	Spending
Total	100.0%	100.0%	100.0%	100.0%	100.0%	100.0%	100.0%	100.0%
Aged	4.4	7.3	2.2	7.3	1.4	1.0	7.1	8.6
Disabled	14.1	28.3	10.0	26.7	15.2	13.0	19.0	41.6
Children	59.6	37.7	62.9	38.1	66.5	52.3	54.7	32.8
Adults	21.8	26.7	24.9	27.9	17.0	33.8	19.1	17.0

Notes: Excludes the territories, Medicaid-expansion CHIP enrollees, and administrative costs. Benefit spending from MSIS data has been adjusted to match CMS-64 totals. Spending is for the respective type of managed care arrangement shown. Children and non-aged adults who qualify for Medicaid on the basis of a disability are included in the disabled category. Enrollees are counted as participating in managed care if at least one managed care payment was made on their behalf during the fiscal year; this method underestimates participation somewhat because it misses enrollees who entered managed care late in the year but for whom a payment was not made until the following fiscal year. Includes federal and state funds. See Section 4 and Tables 11 and 12 in MACStats for more information on how MSIS data used for this table differ from Medicaid Managed Care Enrollment Report data used throughout this Report.

Source: MACPAC analysis of Medicaid Statistical Information System (MSIS) annual person summary (APS) data and CMS-64 Financial Management Report (FMR) net expenditure data from CMS as of May 2011

TABLE B-2. Percentage of Total Medicaid Benefit Spending on Managed Care by Eligibility Group, FY 2008

Basis of Eligibility	Total Medicaid Benefit Spending	Percentage of Total Medicaid Benefit Spending on Managed Care			
		Any managed care	Comprehensive risk-based plans	Primary care case management	Limited-benefit plans
Total	$338.6	21.1%	18.2%	0.3%	2.6%
Aged	70.4	7.4	6.4	0.01	1.1
Disabled	150.5	13.5	10.9	0.1	2.4
Children	68.1	39.6	34.5	0.8	4.2
Adults	49.5	38.6	34.8	0.7	3.0

Notes: Includes federal and state funds. Excludes administrative costs, the territories, and Medicaid-expansion CHIP enrollees. Children and non-aged adults who qualify for Medicaid on the basis of a disability are included in the disabled category. Benefit spending from MSIS data has been adjusted to match CMS-64 totals; see Section 4 of MACStats for methodology.

Source: MACPAC analysis of Medicaid Statistical Information System (MSIS) annual person summary (APS) data and CMS-64 Financial Management Report (FMR) net expenditure data from CMS as of May 2011

small case management fees paid to primary care providers (PCPs). Limited-benefit plans made up 3 percent of all benefit spending in FY 2008.

Beneath this aggregate spending profile, however, patterns differ dramatically by eligibility group. Compared to the average for all of Medicaid, spending on children and adults under age 65—who account for 35 percent of all Medicaid benefit spending (MACStats Figure 3 and Table 7)—is almost twice as likely to go toward managed care payments (21 percent of benefit spending for all groups, 40 to 39 percent for children and adults, respectively).

By contrast, individuals with disabilities under age 65 account for 44 percent of all Medicaid spending (MACStats Figure 3 and Table 7). This group is far less likely to be enrolled in managed care, and only 14 percent of all Medicaid benefit spending for individuals with disabilities went to managed care payments (Table B-2). Medicaid enrollees age 65 and older—representing 21 percent of all Medicaid benefit spending—are the least likely to be enrolled in managed care. Only 7 percent of Medicaid benefit spending for those age 65 and over was for managed care payments.

Opportunities and Challenges in Comprehensive Risk-based Managed Care

When implemented and monitored effectively, comprehensive risk-based Medicaid managed care programs may offer some states opportunities for improving access to and quality of care while potentially constraining program costs. Contracting with plans for comprehensive risk-based managed care may provide states with the ability to require the development of a dedicated network of providers, care management and coordination, and quality measurement standards. How these

goals are achieved may vary by eligibility group, as each one presents opportunities and challenges related to managed care monitoring requirements in contracts. Although some states have chosen to implement PCCM programs or make use of limited-benefit plans alone, this section presents some of the issues that states face when moving enrollees to comprehensive risk-based managed care, then explores how some of these issues are particularly significant for different eligibility groups within Medicaid.

Issues Affecting All Enrollees in Comprehensive Risk-based Plans

Some of the issues that states address in implementing managed care for all Medicaid enrollees in comprehensive risk-based plans include:

- establishing voluntary or mandatory enrollment policies;
- educating enrollees about managed care;
- planning for adequate time to roll-out enrollment for large new populations;
- providing for plan choice and auto-assignment;
- ensuring continuity of care and access to providers;
- setting payment rates in a way that covers the cost of efficiently provided and appropriate care; and
- monitoring plans over time.

Voluntary versus mandatory enrollment. Many states have made enrollment in a comprehensive risk-based managed care plan mandatory for certain populations. Other subgroups of enrollees may be excluded (not eligible for enrollment, sometimes referred to as a population carve out) or exempt (may voluntarily enroll) from mandatory managed care. Some states exclude persons with disabilities, children with special needs, foster children, and medically needy enrollees from enrolling in their managed care program.[4] Carved-out populations either remain in traditional FFS or may be enrolled in a specialized managed care plan with a network of providers that specializes in their specific health care needs (e.g., cystic fibrosis, cancer care, organ transplantation, end-stage renal disease, HIV/AIDS, hemophilia).

When voluntary enrollment in managed care is low, there is the chance that participating plans will not have adequate numbers of enrollees to spread out the risk of high-cost events or to cover certain administrative costs. These issues can be addressed through well-designed payment arrangements. Mandatory enrollment is an approach that has been used to ensure a large number of enrollees participate.

Outreach and enrollee education. When implementing managed care, making sure enrollees understand how managed care works and differs from FFS is a particular concern. For enrollees who have been uninsured or in FFS Medicaid, the enrollment process may be their first interaction with managed care. Thus, when enrolling individuals with Medicaid coverage, it is important to communicate:

- how to obtain services in the most appropriate manner;

- the procedures for making plan selection and the implications of those choices;

- the concept of auto-assignment for those who do not select a plan; and

- the importance of acting in a timely manner so that enrollment cards and new member materials can be issued (Gold et al. 1996).

For Medicaid enrollees, education about the managed care program is crucial. States often contract with enrollment brokers who provide outreach, enrollment, and educational services and serve as a link between managed care plans and enrollees. States may also use community-based organizations to assist enrollees with the enrollment process. States and enrollment brokers often use several strategies to inform enrollees about their managed care choices, including informational materials and instructions on how to enroll, toll-free help lines, and face-to-face counseling.

Roll-out. Successful implementation of Medicaid managed care takes time and may improve with a phased-in roll-out schedule. Implementation must take into consideration adequate time for systems development, as well as sufficient resources to ensure an effective enrollment and transition process for enrollees.

The past experiences of some states that moved quickly to design and implement new managed care programs in the mid-1990s demonstrated the issues that may emerge when rapidly implementing such programs. For example, when Tennessee initially introduced and implemented TennCare in 1994, the state's implementation schedule proved to be too short for adequate preparation by the state and participating managed care plans, including not having operating information systems by the start date of the program. Information and adequate education were not readily available for enrollees who were unfamiliar with managed care concepts; providers were delivering services without knowing whether or by whom they would get paid; and the state was not fully prepared for adequate oversight of the managed care plans (Wooldridge et al. 1996).

---

[4] There are also federal requirements related to the enrollment of American Indians into Medicaid managed care. For example, a state may not require tribal members to enroll in managed care or a PCCM program, except when the entity is the Indian Health Service; an Indian health program operated by a tribe or tribal organization pursuant to a contract, grant, cooperative agreement, or compact with the Indian Health Service; or an urban Indian health program operated by an urban Indian organization pursuant to a grant or contract with the Indian Health Service.

However, this program has matured over the years and now has 93 percent of its Medicaid enrollees in comprehensive risk-based plans (MACStats Table 11).

Plan choice and auto-assignment. For mandatory enrollment in comprehensive risk-based managed care programs, states try to enroll new Medicaid members into a managed care plan as soon as possible after their initial Medicaid eligibility determination. The timing of enrollment in a managed care plan varies across states, with some states requiring enrollees to pick a plan at the time they apply for Medicaid, while other states wait until after Medicaid eligibility has been determined. Thus some Medicaid enrollees may enroll in Medicaid and select a plan at the same time.

Medicaid enrollees are generally offered a choice among health plans and must choose one within a specific window of time (ranging from a number of days to several months, depending on the state). The amount of time may vary by Medicaid subpopulation. For example, some states allow persons with disabilities a longer amount of time to choose a plan compared to non-disabled enrollees. A state that mandates Medicaid managed care enrollment must offer a choice of at least two plans, except in certain rural areas or if the state receives a waiver for this provision (42 CFR 438.52). The number of plans from which Medicaid enrollees may choose can vary by state, county, region, or even by metropolitan area. While some Medicaid enrollees may be offered a choice of 10 managed care plans in a certain area, in other geographic areas they may only be offered two managed care plans. Communicating the differences in managed care plans offered to enrollees is critical for their ability to make informed decisions on which plan best meets their health care needs.

For some individuals, plan enrollment is initiated by a health care encounter. The clinic or hospital providing services often looks into potential eligibility and facilitates enrollment of the individual, if eligible, in Medicaid or CHIP. If the person is in an eligibility category where managed care is mandatory, this enrollment triggers the need to select a plan.

Auto-assignment is a common method of plan selection for enrollees who do not make a choice within the given timeframe. For these enrollees, the state makes the selection and assigns them to a particular health plan. While the methodology for auto-assignment varies across states, federal regulations require that the auto-assignment process try to preserve existing provider-enrollee relationships (42 CFR 438.50). Auto-assignment may also take into consideration the proximity of participating plans and providers, the plan enrollment of other family members, and the balanced distribution of enrollees across plans. Some states use auto-assignment in certain performance-based policies. For example, plans that rank higher on clinical quality outcomes may receive a higher percentage of auto-assigned enrollees. States may also use other factors for auto-assignment. For example, California gives preference in auto-assignment to plans according to their percentage of contracts with safety-net providers and certain performance measures.

Once enrolled in a managed care plan, enrollees often have the ability to switch plans within a certain timeframe (e.g., 90 days from enrollment into plan) without cause. Once the opportunity to switch ends, several states have lock-in provisions that mandate the enrollee stay with the assigned plan for a certain period of time, usually six months or one year.[5]

---

[5] Enrollees may request disenrollment from a plan at least once every 12 months (42 CFR 438.56).

States' capacity to smoothly enroll large populations has been an issue in the past as some states moved to mandatory managed care for large groups. High rates of auto-assignment or plan switching may signal inadequacies in the education and enrollment process. States have offset these problems by modifying enrollment procedures and increasing outreach and education among Medicaid enrollees and providers.

Continuity of care. Another consideration for states when an enrollee transitions from FFS to managed care is the need to minimize disruption in any ongoing course of treatment. States often require plans to allow a transition period during which an enrollee can continue treatment with a given provider for a given period of time, regardless of whether or not the provider is within the plan's network. This helps to ensure continuity of care until the managed care plan can develop a transition plan and identify appropriate providers within the network to meet the enrollees' needs—and also attempt to include the enrollees' provider(s) in the plan's network.

Access to providers. Some states have found it a challenge to secure provider participation in Medicaid, particularly for some specialties, such as behavioral health providers, neurologists, and oncologists. Through contract requirements, states can require managed care plans to develop broad provider networks. As described below, access to specialty care may be a concern for certain populations moving into managed care.

Payment. States must assure that the mechanisms for setting capitation payments to plans are adequate. As states' experience with Medicaid managed care has grown, methods for risk adjusting payments have improved. These considerations are especially important as states move to enroll high cost, high need populations in managed care. More information on payment issues is included in Section D of this Report.

Monitoring. By requiring managed care plans to collect and report ongoing data such as utilization measures, states can ensure that enrollees are receiving continued appropriate access to high-quality services. More information on monitoring access and quality is included in Section E of this Report.

Issues Related to Non-disabled Children and Adults

Non-disabled child and adult Medicaid enrollees under age 65 (such adults often qualify on the basis of being parents of children enrolled in Medicaid) make up 88 percent of the Medicaid enrollees in comprehensive risk-based managed care plans. These two populations are far healthier on average than the rest of the Medicaid population. Nearly three-fourths of children enrolled in Medicaid or CHIP report being in excellent or very good health. This is lower than privately insured children, but higher than adult Medicaid enrollees (MACStats Tables 3B, 4B, 5B).

However, children enrolled in Medicaid and CHIP are not uniformly healthy. About 18 percent of children enrolled in Medicaid and CHIP do not receive SSI benefits but meet the definition of children with special health care needs (CSHCN).[6] On many measures of health status and service use, this group of children is more similar to

---

[6] This definition, used by the federal government and states for policy and program planning purposes and by researchers for analytic purposes, includes children who "have or are at increased risk for a chronic physical, developmental, behavioral, or emotional condition and who also require health and related services of a type or amount beyond that required by children generally." CSHCN encompasses children with disabilities, as well as those with chronic conditions (e.g., asthma, juvenile diabetes, sickle cell anemia) that range from mild to severe. Except for those who are eligible for Medicaid on the basis of a disability, CSHCN are included in the "Children" category throughout this Report. See Section 2 of MACStats for further discussion of the disabled, SSI, and CSHCN populations.

children with disabilities than to other Medicaid/ CHIP children: they are more likely to report fair or poor health status and are nearly twice as likely to visit health care providers four or more times within a year (MACStats Tables 3B and 3C). In managed care statistics available from CMS, non-disabled CSHCN are not tracked separately; they are included in the statistics for all non-disabled children.

Predictable costs. Average benefit spending for non-disabled children in Medicaid was about $3,000 per full-year equivalent enrollee in FY 2008; for non-disabled adults under age 65, average benefit spending was about $4,700 per full-year equivalent enrollee (MACStats Table 8). Spending on individuals with disabilities and enrollees age 65 and older is three to five times as much. Regardless of cost, enrolling various populations in managed care may increase predictability of state spending.

Fluctuations in eligibility. One challenge of managed care for enrolling non-disabled children and adults is fluctuations in their eligibility status. Turnover in program enrollment can be a function of changes in income levels or issues with renewal. An analysis of 2006 Medicaid administrative data indicated non-disabled adults under age 65 had the lowest rates of continuous enrollment and were typically continuously enrolled for just over two-thirds of the year. Individuals age 65 and older and children had rates of continuous enrollment similar to the average, which is three-quarters of the year (Ku et al. 2009).

Interruptions in health care coverage can affect plans' ability to manage and coordinate care for Medicaid enrollees. It can also impair quality monitoring and improvement activities in the provision of health care services. One study found that extending children's enrollment in Medicaid from three months to one year reduced hospitalizations for ambulatory-care-sensitive conditions by about five percent (Bindman et al.

2008). States have used such increases in the period of time between eligibility determinations as one strategy for improving continuity of care. Federal Medicaid policies allow states to provide children with continuous eligibility in the Medicaid program for up to 12 months. As of January 1, 2011, 23 states provided 12-month continuous eligibility in Medicaid programs and 28 states provide it in CHIP (Heberlein et al. 2011).

Adequate provider networks. Enrolling large numbers of children and adults in managed care plans requires that the plans have an adequate network of appropriate providers that can serve the needs of the enrolled populations (42 CFR 438.206). Access to specialists is a particular issue for Medicaid children and adult enrollees. Plans report greater difficulty developing adequate specialty care networks while providers have reported difficulty in making successful referrals for specialty care (Gold et al. 2003).

Pregnant women require a specific set of services and providers for their health care needs. Medicaid provides coverage for pregnant women and their pregnancy-related care, including prenatal, delivery, complications that may occur during pregnancy, and postpartum-related services. Access to adequate obstetrics and gynecology provider networks and prenatal and postnatal services is a component of providing quality care to this population. The cost of care for pregnant women may vary depending on the type of delivery and whether there are any complications. Eligibility determination for this population differs from most other non-disabled adults under age 65 in that pregnant women may become eligible for Medicaid coverage based on their health condition (pregnancy status).

Issues Related to Persons with Disabilities

Persons with disabilities in the Medicaid program are individuals under age 65 (including children) who qualify for federal SSI benefits or meet similar criteria. In most states, qualifying for SSI—a federally funded, cash assistance program for certain low-income aged, blind, and disabled individuals—automatically confers Medicaid eligibility.[7] (For more on SSI eligibility, see Section 4 of MACStats.)

Children receiving SSI represent only 3 percent of non-institutionalized Medicaid/CHIP children under age 19 (MACStats Table 3B). Among non-institutionalized Medicaid adults under age 65, 21 percent receive SSI benefits (MACStats Table 4B). Together, disabled children and adults account for 17 percent of total Medicaid enrollment, but they represent a disproportionate share of program spending (44 percent of total Medicaid benefit spending in FY 2008) (MACStats Tables 6 and 7).

Medicaid enrollees on SSI, both children and adults, report poorer health status and greater presence of health conditions including chronic conditions, compared to the overall Medicaid/ CHIP population in that age group (MACStats Tables 3B and 4B). Over half of Medicaid adults that receive SSI benefits report their health status as fair or poor. Both adults and children on SSI reported more visits to providers within a year, and adults reported more home care within the past 12 months, than other Medicaid/CHIP enrollees in their age group (MACStats Tables 3C and 4C).

In general, persons with disabilities are a high need, high cost group of Medicaid enrollees that can present challenges for managed care, both in terms of service delivery and costs. However, the number of states with SSI enrollees in both voluntary and mandatory managed care has grown over time (GAO 2000).

High cost population. Medicaid benefit spending for persons with disabilities averaged more than $17,000 per full-year equivalent enrollee in FY 2008, the highest of any eligibility group (MACStats Table 8). Cost savings may be a major goal for states implementing managed care for disabled enrollees, but research quantifying state savings from transitioning disabled enrollees into managed care is often limited and narrow in scope; additional data would be helpful.

Despite the potential for savings, the high costs of care for persons with disabilities can also be a barrier to managed care enrollment. Effective setting of payment rates for this population is necessary to protect access to care for high cost enrollees and equity across health plans participating in the program. (For further discussion of Medicaid managed care payment policy, see Section D of this Report).

Stable eligibility. Individuals with disabilities tend to have more stability in their Medicaid eligibility status than non-disabled children and adults under age 65. Individuals with disabilities are more likely to be continuously enrolled than all other Medicaid enrollees, likely reflecting that the income of many of these individuals is stable (Ku et al. 2009).

Voluntary versus mandatory enrollment. Many Medicaid programs that offer managed care to individuals with disabilities have started with voluntary program enrollment. In order for mandatory enrollment to be effective for individuals with disabilities, provider networks

---

[7] Eleven states (Connecticut, Hawaii, Illinois, Indiana, Minnesota, Missouri, New Hampshire, North Dakota, Ohio, Oklahoma, Virginia) known as 209(b) states are allowed to use different financial and non-financial Medicaid eligibility rules from the federal SSI program for Medicaid eligibility determinations as long as the Medicaid rules are no more restrictive than the rules the state had in place in 1972 when the SSI program was enacted.

that take into account the special health care needs of the populations, as well as adequate enrollee education and outreach, are needed.

Continuity of care. Mandatory managed care enrollment of individuals with disabilities has the potential to affect established provider and care arrangements (Tanenbaum and Hurley 1995). Issues of continuity of care may arise for providers and disabled enrollees when a specialty care provider that has developed a relationship with an enrollee is not included in the managed care plan's provider network. This can be further complicated by the fact that enrollees in this group may see a wide variety of providers to address multiple co-morbid conditions. Some states offer a longer transition period for disabled enrollees than they do for managed care enrollees without disabilities, so enrollees can continue ongoing courses of treatment and managed care plans can work to ensure continuity of care. Plans may also choose to allow some enrollees to continue receiving care from an out-of-network provider for a given period of time.

Care coordination. Enrollees with disabilities often have complex medical needs that may require coordination of care across multiple physical and behavioral health providers, as well as pharmacy and dental services. In FFS, management of care is typically the responsibility of the enrollee or the enrollee's family or guardian, though some states provide care coordination services. The care for enrollees with complex chronic conditions may be improved through care management activities.

In well-designed contract provisions states can require managed care plans to coordinate services for enrollees, including scheduling appointments, locating participating providers, helping facilitate communication between providers, identifying health risks, and addressing other issues that may affect access. Plans may also be responsible for providing enrollee education that focuses

on specific health needs, including disease management programs or self-management skills for a particular chronic condition. Well-executed managed care can also focus appropriate attention on care transitions (e.g., hospital to short-term nursing facility to home), which can reduce readmissions to hospitals and nursing facilities, and loss of enrollee long-term independence.

Benefit carve outs can affect care coordination for disabled enrollees. (For further discussion of carved-out benefits see Section C of this Report.) If certain services such as oral health, pharmacy, or behavioral health are carved out of managed care and provided through FFS, enrollees must navigate across multiple environments, and coordination of services becomes more complex. Even for services included in a managed care contract, plans may choose to contract out certain services, which also may raise issues with coordination of care.

Access to care. Medicaid enrollees who qualify for coverage on the basis of a disability have conditions that may include physical impairments and limitations (e.g., quadriplegia), intellectual or developmental impairments (e.g., mental retardation, cerebral palsy), and severe mental and emotional conditions, including mental illness (e.g., schizophrenia). They include children and adults residing in the community, as well as in long-term care facilities. Therefore managed care plans must ensure that their provider network consists of the right types and sufficient numbers of providers to serve this group adequately. States may require plans to allow standing referrals to specialists or designation of a specialist as a PCP.

Issues Related to Persons Dually Eligible for Medicaid and Medicare

Approximately 9 million individuals are dually eligible for Medicare and Medicaid (referred to as "dual eligibles") (MACStats Table 6). These Medicare beneficiaries receive financial assistance from their state Medicaid programs to pay for Medicare premiums, copays and/or deductibles. If their income and assets are low enough, dual eligibles may also qualify for full Medicaid benefits including long-term services and supports (LTSS).

Medicare is the primary payer for dual eligibles, covering all acute care services, outpatient and physician services, dialysis, prescription drugs, and post-acute care services (e.g., rehabilitation following hospitalization). Medicaid "wraps around" Medicare for dual eligibles, paying Medicare premiums and cost sharing (i.e., deductibles and copays) and covering services with limited or no Medicare coverage including LTSS, behavioral health, and medical transportation services.

Dual eligibles can be enrolled in varying combinations of FFS and managed care for their Medicare and Medicaid benefits. These combinations can vary by state and within market areas of individual states. Most dual eligibles, however, currently receive care for Medicare and Medicaid services in FFS settings.

High cost population. Spending on dual eligibles varies substantially according to health status, physical and cognitive impairments, and whether or not they reside in an institution. Medicaid and Medicare per enrollee spending on dual eligibles totaled $26,185 in 2005 with Medicaid spending accounting for 63 percent of the total (MedPAC 2010).[8] Dual eligibles' Medicare spending is also higher than for the average Medicare beneficiary. This has created an interest in finding better ways to coordinate and manage care for this population in both programs.

Voluntary versus mandatory managed care. For services covered by Medicare, federal law requires that a beneficiary's enrollment in managed care must be voluntary (§1802 of the Social Security Act). Incentives for dual eligibles to join Medicare managed care plans, known as Medicare Advantage (MA) plans, may be limited because some of the additional benefits and reduced cost sharing that MA plans offer to attract enrollees are already covered by Medicaid. Approximately 1.5 million dual eligibles—less than 20 percent of this population—have exercised the option to enroll in an MA plan for their Medicare benefits (Bella and Palmer 2009).

A larger number of dual eligibles—over 2 million—are enrolled in some form of managed care for their Medicaid benefits (CMS 2010). State policies determine whether dual eligibles have the option to enroll in Medicaid managed care, whether enrollment is voluntary or mandatory, and whether certain services such as behavioral health and LTSS are provided by the managed care plan or through FFS. States may also establish policies regarding simultaneous enrollment in Medicare and Medicaid managed care plans and whether dual eligibles can receive both program benefits from the same health plan or from two separate health plans (Walsh 2002).

Integrating Medicare and Medicaid. Medicare and Medicaid have different statutory provisions, administrative procedures, and payment policies, which can complicate coordination of services and payments. States, CMS, and health plans also jointly face challenges in effectively sharing information.

---

[8] The data predate the implementation of Medicare's drug benefit so prescription drug spending is included in Medicaid's spending.

For dual eligibles in managed care, Medicare and Medicaid services and benefits may be coordinated to different degrees under current law. Examples include:

▶ an MA plan with Medicaid FFS "wrap around" for acute care cost sharing and coverage of LTSS;

▶ an MA plan (possibly a Special Needs Plan (SNP)) and a companion Medicaid managed care plan with a primary, acute, and LTSS contract; and

▶ a fully integrated provider-based managed care plan that provides all Medicare and Medicaid primary and acute care services and LTSS. The Program of All-Inclusive Care for the Elderly (PACE) is a model of fully integrated Medicare and Medicaid services and financing for dual eligibles.

SNPs. SNPs are MA plans that focus on certain groups of Medicare enrollees. There are three types of SNPs: SNPs for dual eligibles (D-SNPs), SNPs for Medicare enrollees with severe or disabling chronic conditions (C-SNPs), and SNPs for Medicare beneficiaries in institutions such as nursing homes (I-SNPs). SNPs are able to target or limit plan enrollment to these specific subsets of the Medicare population.

As of April 2011, 298 D-SNPs were operating with an enrollment of approximately 1.1 million (CMS 2011a). Full integration of Medicare and Medicaid benefits requires the D-SNP to have a contract with the state for the provision of Medicaid benefits, in addition to an MA contract. Most D-SNPs currently do not have contracts with states to provide full Medicaid benefits. Only an estimated 120,000 dual eligibles, or less than 1.5 percent of the total dual eligible population, are enrolled in fully integrated managed care programs (Bella and Palmer 2009).

In an effort to improve the integration of Medicare and Medicaid benefits, the Medicare Improvements for Patients and Providers Act of 2008 (MIPPA, P.L. 110-275, §164) mandates that new D-SNPs, or existing D-SNPs seeking to expand into new service areas, must enter into contractual relationships with states to provide Medicaid benefits for D-SNP enrollees. The regulations authorizing contracting requirements (42 CFR 422.107) have offered some additional guidelines on this requirement, detailing what must be contained in the contract between the state and the D-SNP, including the MA organization's responsibilities (e.g., financial obligations) to provide or arrange for Medicaid benefits, Medicaid benefits covered under the SNP, and cost-sharing protections.

PACE. The PACE program is a provider-based model for qualifying frail elderly dual eligibles that integrates Medicare and Medicaid services and financing. PACE programs—which are offered by nonprofit or public entities—provide social and medical services primarily in an adult day health center, supplemented by in-home and referral services in accordance with the enrollee's needs. The PACE model of care is a permanent provision within the Medicare program, but an option for state Medicaid programs. States must include PACE as an optional Medicaid benefit in their state Medicaid plan before the state and the Secretary of the Department of Health and Human Services (HHS) can enter into program agreements with PACE providers. Currently 82 PACE organizations in 30 states have enrolled approximately 20,000 dual eligibles (CMS 2011a).

Acting as the sole source of services for enrollees, PACE providers assume full financial risk for participants' care without limits on amount, duration, or scope of services. PACE providers receive separate monthly Medicare and Medicaid capitation payments for each eligible enrollee. Under the Medicare program, the standard risk-adjusted capitation rate that CMS pays to MA plans is adjusted to include an additional patient frailty adjustment for PACE enrollees. The monthly Medicaid capitation rate is negotiated between the PACE provider and the state agency and is specified in the contract between them. This Medicaid capitation rate is fixed during the contract year regardless of changes in the enrollee's health status.

Evaluations of PACE programs have found them to be a successful model of care for frail elderly individuals, in terms of several measures of outcomes, including health and functional status, qualify of life, and satisfaction with services (Chatterji et al. 1998). However, only about 10 percent of eligible individuals choose to enroll in PACE. Additionally, the availability of PACE programs is limited in many parts of the country, due in part to the high start-up costs to develop new delivery sites and the financial risk for organizations that choose to establish PACE programs. Some organizations are exploring the concept of "PACE without walls," which would provide options for integration of acute and LTSS in the community without the need for a single "bricks and mortar" delivery site.

CMS Activities and Demonstrations. The new Federal Coordinated Health Care Office (FCHCO) at CMS, created by the Patient Protection and Affordable Care Act (P.L. 111-148, §2602), is intended to work toward integrating care for dual eligibles and coordinating benefits between Medicaid and Medicare. FCHCO recently published a list of areas in which the two programs could better align their requirements, including coordinated care, FFS benefits, prescription drugs, cost sharing, enrollment, and appeals (CMS 2011b).

On April 14, 2011, CMS announced 15 states selected to receive design contracts as part of the agency's initiative on State Demonstrations to Integrate Care for Dual Eligible Individuals.[9] Each state will receive up to $1 million to design a delivery system and payment model to improve coordination of care across primary, acute, behavioral health, and LTSS for dual eligibles. States that successfully complete their design may be eligible to receive additional funding to implement their proposals.

---

[9] The states selected were California, Colorado, Connecticut, Massachusetts, Michigan, Minnesota, New York, North Carolina, Oklahoma, Oregon, South Carolina, Tennessee, Vermont, Washington, and Wisconsin.

References

Bella, M., and L. Palmer. 2009. *Encouraging Integrated Care for Dual Eligibles.* Hamilton, NJ: Center for Health Care Strategies (CHCS), Inc. http://www.chcs.org/usr_doc/Integrated_Care_Resource_Paper.pdf.

Bindman, A.B. , A. Chattopadhyay, and G.M. Auerback. 2008. Medicaid re-enrollment policies and children's risk of hospitalizations for ambulatory care sensitive conditions. *Medical Care* 46, no. 10: 1049–1054.

Centers for Medicare & Medicaid Services (CMS), Department of Health and Human Services. 2011a. Communication with MACPAC.

Centers for Medicare & Medicaid Services (CMS), Department of Health and Human Services. 2011b. Medicare and Medicaid programs; Opportunities for alignment under Medicaid and Medicare. *Federal Register* 76, No. 94: 28196-28207. http://www.cms.gov/medicare-medicaid-coordination/Downloads/FederalRegisterNoticeforComment052011.pdf.

Centers for Medicare & Medicaid Services (CMS), Department of Health and Human Services. 2010. *Medicaid Managed care enrollment report.* https://www.cms.gov/MedicaidDataSourcesGenInfo/04_MdManCrEnrllRep.asp.

Centers for Medicare & Medicaid Services (CMS), Department of Health and Human Services. 2008. Annual person summary MSIS File.

Centers for Medicare & Medicaid Services (CMS), Department of Health and Human Services. 2005. Annual person summary MSIS File.

Chatterji, P., N. Burstein, D. Kidder, A. White. 1998. *Evaluation of the Program of All-Inclusive Care for the Elderly (PACE) Demonstration: The impact if PACE on participant outcomes.* Report to the Health Care Financing Administration (now CMS). Cambridge, MA: Abt Associates. http://www.cms.gov/DemoProjectsEvalRpts/downloads/PACE_Outcomes.pdf.

Gold M., J. Mittler, D. Draper, and D. Rousseau. 2003. Participation of plans and providers in Medicaid and SCHIP managed care. *Health Affairs* 22, no. 1: 230-240.

Gold, M., M. Sparer, and K. Chu. 1996. Medicaid managed care for low-income populations: Lessons from five states. *Health Affairs* 15, no. 3: 153-166.

Government Accountability Office (GAO). 2000. *Challenges in implementing safeguards for children with special needs.* http://www.gao.gov/new.items/he00037.pdf.

Heberlein, M., T. Brooks, J. Guyer, et al. 2011. *Holding steady, looking ahead: Annual findings of a 50-state survey of eligibility rules, enrollment and renewal procedures, and cost sharing practices in Medicaid and CHIP, 2010-2011.* Washington, DC: Kaiser Commission on Medicaid and the Uninsured. http://www.kff.org/medicaid/upload/8130.pdf.

Ku, L., P. MacTaggart, F. Pervez, and S. Rosenbaum. 2009. *Improving Medicaid's continuity of coverage and quality of care. Report to the Association for Community Affiliated Plans.* Washington, DC: George Washington University Department of Health Policy. http://www.ahcahp.org/Portals/0/ACAP%20Docs/Improving%20Medicaid%20Final%20070209.pdf.

Ku, L., M. Ellwood, S. Hoag, B. Ormond, and J. Wooldridge. 2000. Evolution of Medicaid managed care systems and eligibility expansions. *Health Care Financing Review* 22, no.2: 7-27.

Medicaid and CHIP Payment and Access Commission (MACPAC). March 2011. *Report to the Congress on Medicaid and CHIP.* Washington, DC: MACPAC. March 2011. http://www.macpac.gov/reports/MACPAC_March2011_web.pdf.

Medicare Payment Advisory Commission (MedPAC). 2010. Coordinating the care of dual eligible beneficiaries. In *Report to the Congress: Aligning Incentives in Medicare. Chapter 5.* Washington, DC: MedPAC. http://www.medpac.gov/chapters/Jun10_Ch05.pdf.

Rowland, D., and B Lyons. 1987. Mandatory HMO care for Milwaukee's poor. *Health Affairs* 6, no.1: 87-100.

Tanenbaum, S., and R. Hurley. 1995. Disability and the managed care frenzy: A cautionary note. *Health Affairs* 14, no. 4: 213-219.

Walsh, E., and W. Clark. 2002. Managed care and dually eligible beneficiaries: Challenges in coordination. *Health Care Financing Review* 24, no. 1: 63-82.

Wooldridge J., L. Ku, T. Coughlin, L. Dubay, M. Ellwood, S. Rajan, S. Hoag, 1996. *Implementing state health care reform: What have we learned from the first year? The First Annual Report of the Evaluation of Health Reform in Five States.* Washington, DC: Mathematica Policy Research, Inc. http://www.mathematica-mpr.com/publications/PDFs/health/implementstatehealth.pdf.

SECTION

Managed Care Plans

The term "managed care" in Medicaid is used to refer to a broad spectrum of arrangements. In addition to comprehensive risk-based managed care plans, which are most like private health maintenance organizations (HMOs), CMS also includes primary care case management (PCCM) programs and limited-benefit plans in the agency's classification of Medicaid managed care. Use of these arrangements varies within and across states, as do the specific service delivery characteristics of each model and the maturity of each state's program. This variation presents challenges in making comparisons across states and Medicaid managed care arrangements. (See the Annex to this section for descriptions of Medicaid managed care terms used throughout this Report.)

States vary on which benefits they include or exclude from their managed care programs. States often carve out or exclude certain Medicaid services from the set of benefits that a comprehensive risk-based managed care plan is responsible for providing to enrollees. These excluded services tend to be provided under fee-for-service (FFS) arrangements or through limited-benefit plans. While states operate their managed care programs under a broad federal framework (described in greater detail in Section F of this Report), the level of detail of requirements that is included in managed care contracts between the state and the plan also varies considerably.

This section describes:

- the types of managed care arrangements used by states;
- the characteristics of managed care plans participating in Medicaid; and
- benefits that are commonly carved out of comprehensive risk-based managed care plans.

Types of Medicaid Managed Care Arrangements

Three main types of managed care arrangements are used by state Medicaid programs today: comprehensive risk-based managed care, PCCM, and limited-benefit plans.

Comprehensive risk-based managed care. In comprehensive risk-based arrangements, states contract with managed care plans to cover all or most Medicaid-covered services for their Medicaid enrollees. Plans are paid a capitation rate, which is a fixed amount per member per month to cover a defined set of services for a given population. While plans are responsible for providing or arranging for a majority of an enrollee's medical needs, the state's obligation to Medicaid enrollees still exists. Plans are at financial risk if spending on benefits and administration exceeds payments; conversely they are permitted to retain any portion of payments not expended for covered services and other contractually required activities. The level of risk for plans varies from state to state and across covered populations within states (for more on risk arrangements, see Section D of this Report). Sometimes one or more benefits, such as behavioral health services, oral health services, non-emergency transportation, or prescription drugs are "carved out" and provided separately through FFS arrangements or by limited-benefit plans.

PCCM. An alternative to comprehensive risk-based arrangements is PCCM, in which enrollees have a single designated primary care provider (PCP) who is paid a monthly case management fee to assume responsibility for enrollee care management and coordination. Individual providers are not at financial risk in PCCM programs; they continue to be paid on an FFS basis for providing covered services. Several states have enhanced their PCCM programs by adding additional coordinated care management features.

These features provide intensive care management for enrollees with high levels of need, increasing their use of performance and quality measures, and providing practice support for individual providers (Verdier et al. 2009). In some cases, financial incentives for both PCPs and the care management entity have also been added.

Limited-benefit Plans. Some states have contracts to manage a subset of benefits (e.g., transportation, oral health services) or services for a particular subpopulation (e.g., individuals in need of inpatient mental health services). These limited-benefit plans are generally paid on a capitated basis and may be risk-based. They may be used to provide a certain set of services to either FFS enrollees, managed care enrollees or both. For purposes of this Report, Prepaid Inpatient Health Plans (PIHPs) and Prepaid Ambulatory Health Plans (PAHPs) are defined as limited-benefit plans. As defined in federal regulation (42 CFR 438.2):

- **PIHPs** cover, among other services, inpatient hospital and institutional services. Such plans most frequently focus on providing inpatient mental health or combined mental health and substance abuse inpatient benefits.

- **PAHPs** are generally very narrow in service scope, typically covering just one type of service. States most commonly use PAHPs to provide only transportation benefits. Other PAHPs may provide oral health services, non-institutional mental health benefits, or disease management.

Table C-1 outlines features associated with various service delivery and payment models, including FFS, comprehensive risk-based managed care, PCCM, and limited-benefit plans.

Seventy-one percent of all Medicaid enrollees received at least some kind of service through managed care, as defined by CMS, in 2009—including comprehensive-risk based managed

TABLE C-1. Overview of Medicaid FFS and Medicaid Managed Care Arrangements[1]

Key System Features	FFS	Comprehensive Risk-based Plans	PCCM Programs	Limited-benefit Plans[2]
Provider participation requirements	Any willing provider licensed by the state who agrees to accept Medicaid rates as payment in full can participate.	Plans must meet network size and location standards. Plans are permitted to limit the number of providers in their network and generally must credential providers before accepting them into the network.	PCCM programs may have to meet additional state requirements and agree to certain service policies.	Plans contract with a network of providers, similar to the process for comprehensive risk-based managed care plans, and may also need to meet network requirements.
Enrollee care-seeking rules	Typically, enrollees may receive care from any participating provider.	Plans set the rules on nonemergency referrals and care management, subject to state requirements and oversight. Services must be received from participating network providers, except in emergencies.	Enrollees may need referral by the PCP to see various kinds of specialists, except in emergencies.	Plans set the rules on nonemergency referrals and care management, subject to state requirements and oversight. Services typically must be received from participating network providers, except in emergencies.
Navigation support for enrollees	Open access; enrollees may or may not not have rules or guidance on how or where to seek appropriate available services.	Plans typically must provide enrollees with a member handbook and conduct an initial health assessment to determine enrollee needs. Many also provide disease management and care coordination services.	PCCM programs may provide additional navigation support and ways of identifying appropriate providers.	Depending on the type of services provided, plans may provide navigation support for enrollees similar to comprehensive risk-based plans.
Performance monitoring and quality oversight	Provider accountability for outcomes for individual enrollees is not typically formalized. For example, most states do not require providers to report HEDIS data.[3]	Plans must conduct external quality reviews and must report specific performance data (e.g., HEDIS) and undertake specific quality improvement activities. Some states require external accreditation (e.g., NCQA and URAC).[4]	Same as FFS; potentially specific metrics associated with monitoring PCCM performance.	PIHPs must conduct annual external quality reviews, may be required to report performance data applicable to the services delivered, and undertake specific quality improvement activities.[5] External accreditation may be required.

Source: MACPAC analysis

[1] Some states have contracted with vendors to administer elements of their programs. Known as administrative services organizations (ASOs), these vendors are typically paid a non-risk-based fee to provide administrative services. While not defined within federal statute or regulations, depending on how they are structured, ASOs may or may not be classified as a managed care arrangement.

[2] Limited-benefit plans may have all, some, or none of the elements of the key system features listed above, depending on the benefits covered and type of contracting arrangement with a state. For example, state contracts with limited-benefit plans for providing behavioral health or oral health services may include requirements regarding network development, assistance to enrollees seeking services and development of member materials.

[3] HEDIS is Healthcare Effectiveness Data and Information Set.

[4] NCQA is National Committee for Quality Assurance, and URAC (formerly known as the Utilization Review Accreditation Commission).

[5] PAHPs are not required to conduct an external quality review.

FIGURE C-1. **Percentage of Medicaid Enrollees In Managed Care Arrangements Nationwide, 2009**

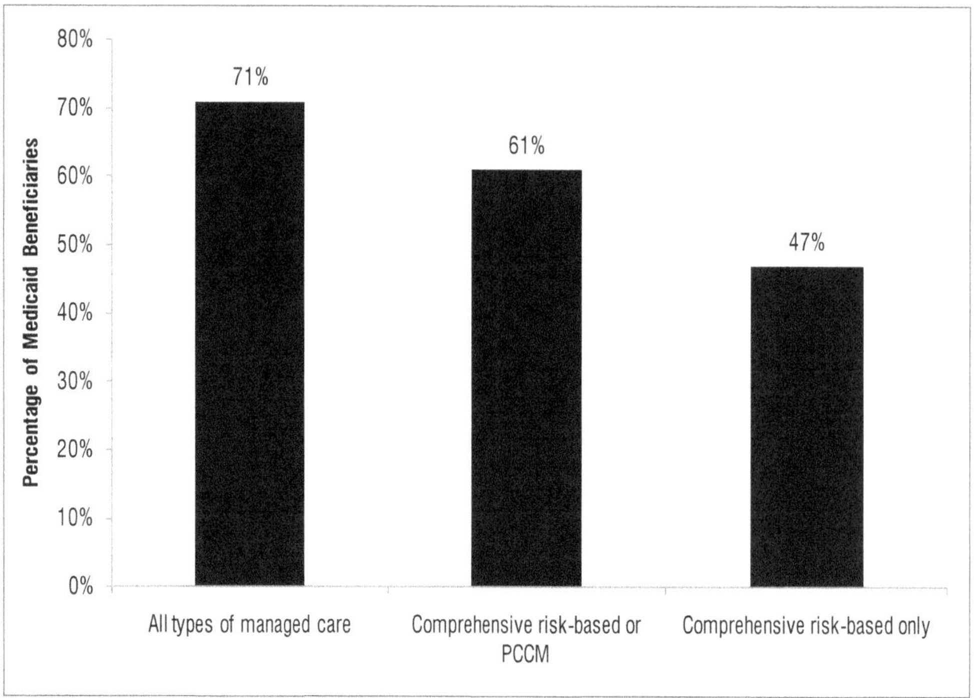

Notes: Includes CHIP enrollees in Medicaid-expansion programs but not in stand-alone programs. U.S. territories are excluded. MACPAC's estimate of national managed care enrollment (71 percent) differs from that reported by CMS (72 percent) due to the exclusion of the territories. The comprehensive risk-based or PCCM "unrounded" number is 61.47% and is reported as 61%. Comprehensive risk-based includes plans categorized by CMS as commercial managed care plans, Medicaid-only plans, Health Insuring Organizations (HIOs), and Programs of All-Inclusive Care for the Elderly (PACE). HIOs exist only in California where selected county-authorized health systems serve Medicaid enrollees. PACE programs combine Medicare and Medicaid financing for qualifying frail elderly dual eligibles.

Source: MACStats Table 9

care, PCCM, and limited-benefit plans (Figure C-1, MACStats Table 9).[6] Excluding the limited-benefit plans results in a nationwide enrollment of 61 percent in either a comprehensive risk-based plan or a PCCM program, with 47 percent of enrollees in a comprehensive risk-based plan only.[7] There is wide variation in the types of plans offered across states (MACStats Table 10).

Comprehensive Risk-based Plans

States have increasingly relied upon comprehensive risk-based managed care when delivering care to Medicaid enrollees. As Figure C-2 shows, 15 percent of Medicaid enrollees were in a comprehensive risk-based arrangement in 1995. By 2009 almost half were in a comprehensive risk-based plan.[8]

---

[6] Of the U.S. territories and Puerto Rico, managed care data are collected only for Puerto Rico and the U.S. Virgin Islands. Based on these available data, only Puerto Rico includes Medicaid managed care in its benefit design.

[7] The CMS Medicaid managed care enrollment statistics include CHIP enrollees who are covered through Medicaid-expansion programs but not enrollees in separate, stand-alone CHIP programs. CMS reported a combined enrollment in managed care plans across all states and plan types of 48.8 million. An analysis of the CMS enrollment data by plan type shows an unduplicated count of 35.2 million enrollees in 2009. The duplicated count exceeded the unduplicated count by about 13 million or 38 percent. Some states have particularly high ratios of unduplicated to duplicated counts, indicating that on average Medicaid enrollees are in more than one type of managed care. This seems to reflect the large limited-benefit program enrollments in states that also have other forms of managed care.

[8] MACPAC's estimate of comprehensive risk-based enrollment (47 percent) differs from that reported by CMS (48 percent) due to the exclusion of the U.S. territories.

FIGURE C-2. Percentage of Medicaid Enrollees in Medicaid Managed Care by Arrangement Type, 1995 and 2000–2009 (excludes limited-benefit plans)

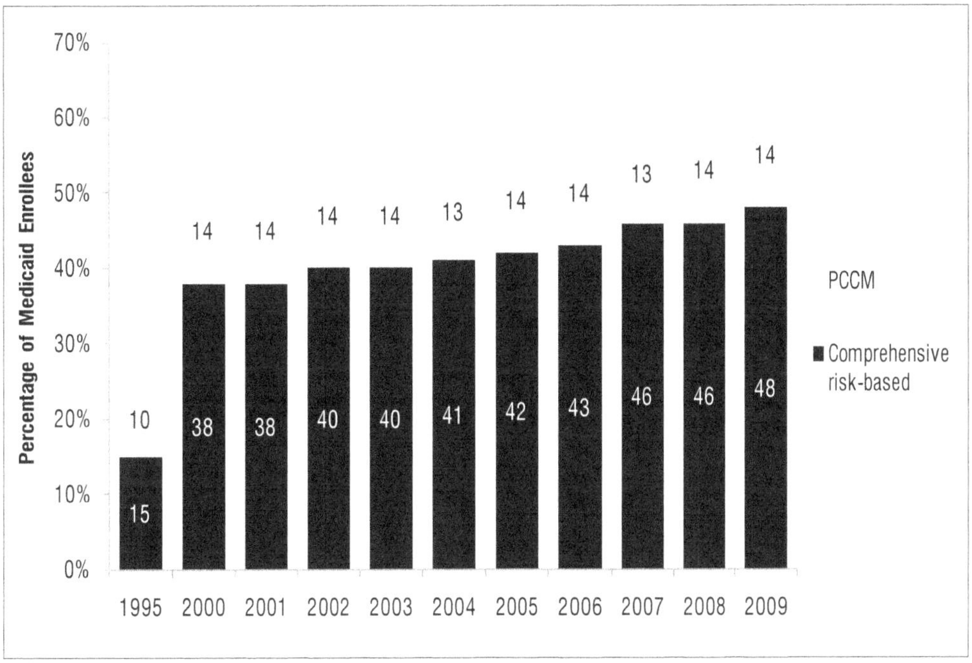

Notes: Includes CHIP enrollees in Medicaid-expansion programs but not in stand-alone programs. Includes Puerto Rico and the U.S. Virgin Islands. The estimate of comprehensive risk-based and PCCM enrollment in Figure C-1 and throughout this Report (47 percent and 61 percent) differs from the figure shown here (48 percent and 62 percent) due to the exclusion of the U.S. territories. Comprehensive risk-based includes plans categorized by CMS as commercial managed care plans, Medicaid-only plans, Health Insuring Organizations (HIOs), and Programs of All-Inclusive Care for the Elderly (PACE). HIOs exist only in California where selected county-authorized health systems serve Medicaid enrollees. PACE programs combine Medicare and Medicaid financing for qualifying frail elderly dual eligibles.

Source: Calculated from CMS Medicaid Managed Care Enrollment Report Summary Statistics, various years

Figure C-3 shows the percentage of Medicaid enrollment in comprehensive risk-based managed care across the states. The 21 states (plus the District of Columbia) with more than half of their Medicaid populations in comprehensive risk-based managed care were mainly concentrated in the East Coast, West Coast, and the upper Midwest. Nine states have no enrollment in comprehensive risk-based managed care.[9] Several others have only a small share of enrollees in such programs: Colorado (10 percent), Illinois (8 percent), Kentucky (21 percent), and Nebraska (17 percent).

PCCM Programs

As shown in Figure C-4, 30 states operated PCCM programs in 2009, with a total enrollment of 7.3 million. Eleven of those states had no enrollment in comprehensive risk-based plans. Nineteen states with comprehensive risk-based managed care arrangements also had PCCM programs. For example, some states have used PCCM in rural areas when they have had difficulties attracting and retaining comprehensive risk-based plans to serve those areas. The eight states that had more than 50 percent of their

[9] Seven states (Arkansas, Iowa, Louisiana, Montana, North Carolina, North Dakota, and Oklahoma) have very small PACE programs. Per CMS, Utah has comprehensive risk-based plans that are regulated as PIHPs.

FIGURE C-3.   Percentage of Medicaid Enrollment in Comprehensive Risk-based Plans by State, 2009

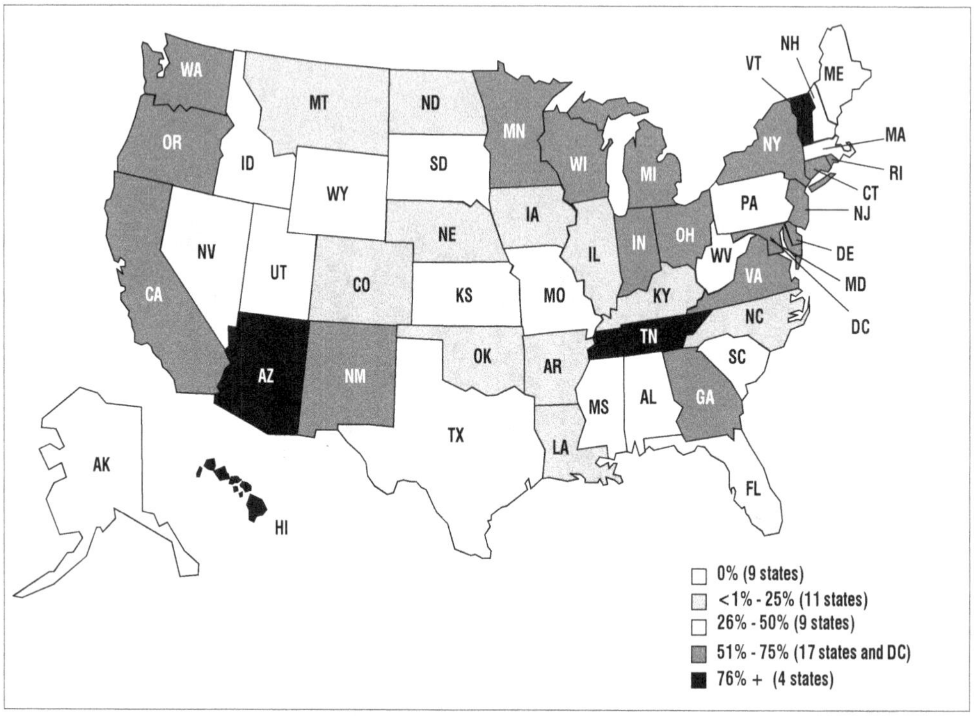

Legend:
- 0% (9 states)
- <1% - 25% (11 states)
- 26% - 50% (9 states)
- 51% - 75% (17 states and DC)
- 76% + (4 states)

Note: Includes CHIP enrollees in Medicaid expansion-programs but not in stand-alone programs. Comprehensive risk-based includes plans categorized by CMS as commercial managed care plans, Medicaid-only plans, Health Insuring Organizations (HIOs), and the Program of All-Inclusive Care for the Elderly (PACE). HIOs exist only in California where Medicaid supports selected county-authorized health systems. The PACE program combines Medicare and Medicaid financing for qualifying frail elderly dual eligibles. See MACStats Table 9 for additional information.

Source: MACPAC analysis of CMS 2009 Medicaid Managed Care Enrollment Report Summary Statistics as of June 30, 2009

enrollment in PCCM programs in 2009 had no comprehensive risk-based plan enrollment (MACStats Table 9).

Limited-benefit Plans

Thrity-four states and the District of Columbia have limited-benefit plan arrangements. Creating an unduplicated count of how many enrollees are served by these plans is challenging, because some states use limited-benefit plans to cover more than one service. According to CMS, there are 8.6 million Medicaid enrollees in PIHPs and 7.9 million enrollees in PAHPs. There are 4.3 million enrollees in PIHPs covering inpatient mental health services; 3.1 million enrollees are in

PIHPs that provide combined mental health and substance abuse benefits; 6.1 million are in PAHPs that provided transportation services only; and 1.2 million are in dental PAHPs.

Characteristics of Comprehensive Risk-based Medicaid Managed Care Plans

The evolution in the Medicaid managed care market over the past 20 years has made it difficult to compare policies and plan types across states. However, comprehensive risk-based Medicaid managed care plans can be classified in a number

FIGURE C-4. Percentage of Medicaid Enrollment in PCCM by State, 2009

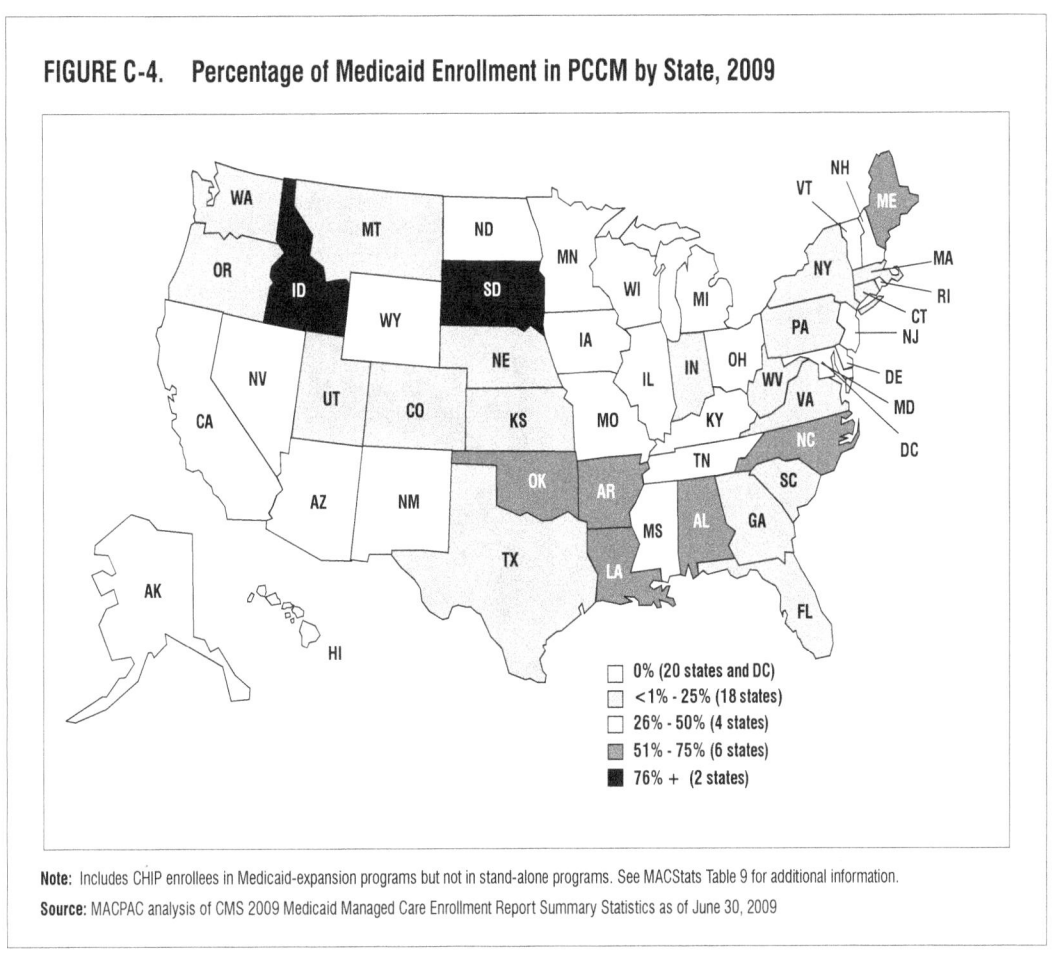

Legend:
- 0% (20 states and DC)
- <1% - 25% (18 states)
- 26% - 50% (4 states)
- 51% - 75% (6 states)
- 76% + (2 states)

Note: Includes CHIP enrollees in Medicaid-expansion programs but not in stand-alone programs. See MACStats Table 9 for additional information.

Source: MACPAC analysis of CMS 2009 Medicaid Managed Care Enrollment Report Summary Statistics as of June 30, 2009

of ways, including whether or not they operate in one or multiple states and how they are sponsored.

Variation among plans includes the extent to which they have enrollees who are insured in the commercial market or Medicare, in addition to Medicaid enrollees.[10] In the mid-to-late 1990s, Medicaid participation by commercial health plans declined, leaving Medicaid more dependent on Medicaid-dominant plans (Felt-Lisk et al. 2001). The Balanced Budget Act of 1997 (BBA, P.L. 105-

33) intensified this trend by eliminating the OBRA 1981 "75/25" rule that required comprehensive risk-based Medicaid managed care plans to have at least 25 percent of their enrollment in the private insurance market. This policy change made it easier for plans to participate in Medicaid. Recent data on the relative performance of different types of Medicaid managed care plans are limited, with many studies dating from the period just after the elimination of the "75/25" rule.

[10] In its 2010 Medicaid Managed Care Enrollment Data Dictionary for the Medicaid Managed Care Data Collection System, CMS uses the term "commercial" to refer to plans that provide comprehensive services to privately insured enrollees and/or Medicare enrollees. CMS uses the term "Medicaid-only" for plans that provide comprehensive services to only Medicaid enrollees, not to commercial or Medicare enrollees. As many Medicaid managed care plans participate in Medicaid as well as CHIP and other public programs, the term "Medicaid-dominant" plans more accurately captures these plans that primarily serve enrollees in these programs.

FIGURE C-5.   Medicaid Managed Care Enrollment Market Share by Firm, 2009

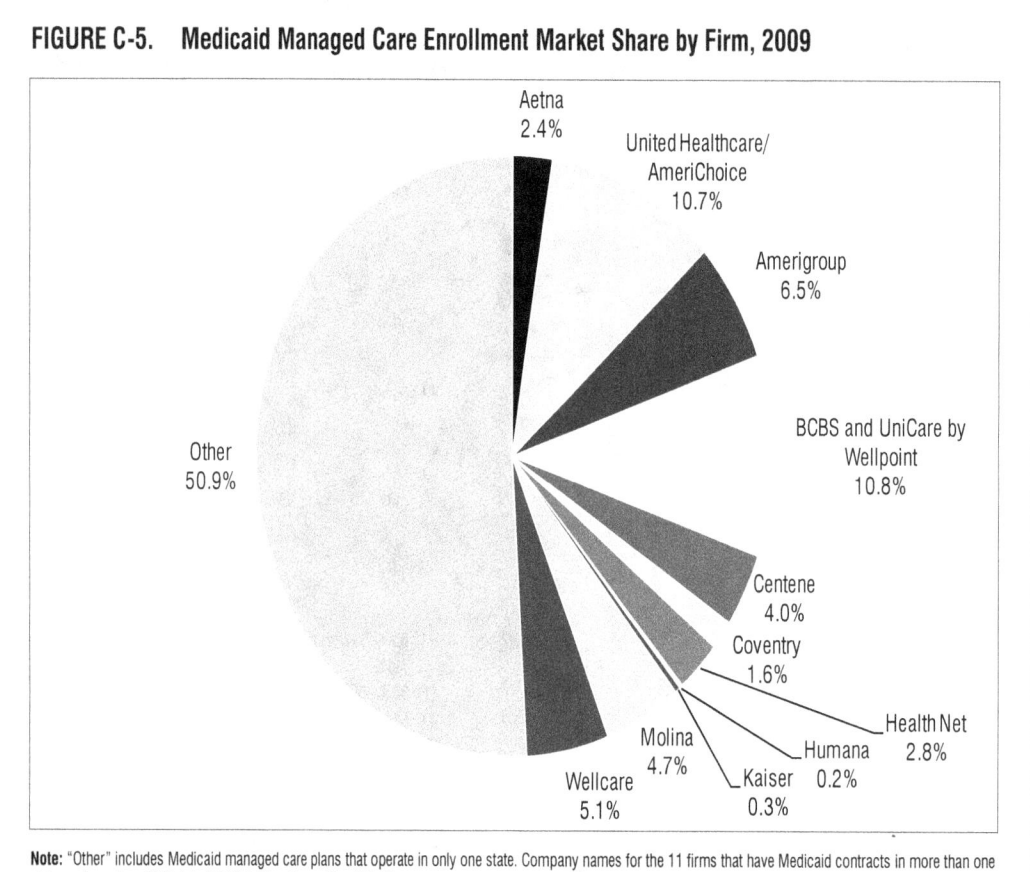

Note: "Other" includes Medicaid managed care plans that operate in only one state. Company names for the 11 firms that have Medicaid contracts in more than one state are based on CMS data. BCBS is Blue Cross/Blue Shield.

Source: MACPAC analysis of CMS 2009 Medicaid Managed Care Enrollment Report Summary Statistics as of June 30, 2009

Plans also vary in their geographic scope. About half (49 percent) of enrollees in comprehensive risk-based Medicaid managed care in 2009 were in plans that operated in multiple states. As shown in Figure C-5, these 11 national firms in 2009 included companies active in the commercial insurance market such as Wellpoint and United Healthcare, as well as firms that have historically focused on the Medicaid market, such as Molina and Centene.[11]

Fifty-one percent of Medicaid enrollees in comprehensive risk-based managed care were enrolled in plans that operated within a single state or region within a state. In addition to commercial plans that operate in a single state or region, these types of plans also include:

▸ Provider-sponsored plans that are typically based around providers such as safety-net hospitals or community health centers that tend to have a history of serving low-income populations. Medicaid is an important payer for many of these plans, who also serve as safety net providers for uninsured individuals.

---

[11] Company names are based on CMS Medicaid Managed Care Enrollment data.

> Government-sponsored plans are created by state and local governments to provide managed care to Medicaid enrollees in a given geographical area. Established as independent health authorities to provide more local control and administration, these plans may constitute a single delivery system for all Medicaid enrollees in the jurisdiction or they may coexist and compete with other health plans in the area.

Carving Out of Comprehensive Risk-based Plan Benefit Packages

In administering their Medicaid managed care programs, states decide which benefits are the responsibility of the managed care plan and which populations are required to enroll, may voluntarily enroll, or are excluded from managed care. States often choose to "carve out" certain services or subpopulations of enrollees from comprehensive risk-based managed care. What services are carved out varies substantially across states depending on how states' Medicaid benefits are structured and provider systems are organized and financed.

States are increasingly looking to managed care to serve not only low-income children and families, but also enrollees with more complex health needs who have often been carved out of comprehensive risk-based managed care in the past. Issues such as coordination of care and system navigation will be important considerations when determining if certain services or populations should be carved out of managed care. In this section we address service carve outs. In Section B of this Report we address population carve outs.

Considerations for Carving Services Out of Comprehensive Risk-based Managed Care

States can choose to carve out certain Medicaid services from a managed care benefit package and provide the excluded benefits under FFS arrangements or through limited-benefit plans specific to that type of service. When services are carved out of the managed care benefit package, the health plan does not receive payment for, nor does it have the responsibility to provide these services. Behavioral health services tend to be the most commonly carved out services in Medicaid programs. Other common carve outs include oral health services, pharmacy services, and nonemergency transportation benefits.

There are many issues for states to consider with regard to carve outs:

Economies of scale and administration. Some benefits, such as transportation, may be more economical when provided directly by the state or through a single, competitively bid contract. Using a single pharmacy benefit manager may make it easier for providers to know what the state formulary covers rather than working with the formularies of multiple Medicaid managed care plans. On the other hand, carve outs may lead to inappropriate provision of care, particularly when one of the services which is a substitute for the other is not included in the plan. (Blumenthal and Buntin 1998).

Fiscal considerations. There may be financial considerations that influence states' decisions to carve out certain services. For example, the Medicaid Drug Rebate Program, which was established in the Omnibus Budget Reconciliation Act of 1990 (P.L. 101-508), helps lower Medicaid spending on outpatient prescription drugs. Originally, rebates were extended only to drugs provided through

FFS Medicaid, not through managed care. To ensure they got the full benefit of the statutory Medicaid rebate, many states carved out pharmacy benefits from their managed care benefit packages.

Effective March 23, 2010, the Patient Protection and Affordable Care Act (P.L. 111-148) extended the Medicaid Drug Rebate Program to managed care plans in Medicaid. As a result of this legislative change, some states (including Texas and New York) are now considering adding pharmacy benefits into their managed care contracts rather than carving them out (NY 2011, TX 2011).

▷ **Quality.** Depending on the structure of the carve out and level of coordination, carve-out arrangements have the potential to improve access to and quality of care by facilitating enrollee access. On the other hand, carve outs have the potential to make it harder to coordinate the services that are carved out with other health services used by enrollees. For example, in some states, behavioral health services are carved out of the plan benefit package but the plan remains responsible for the pharmaceutical costs related to behavioral health. This makes it challenging for plans to coordinate with prescribing providers and to gain a full picture of their enrollees' health needs. Sharing data with comprehensive risk-based plans around carved-out services can assist with care coordination and disease management.

Research on the impact of carve outs on quality and access is limited, and results are mixed. Depending on the service, certain studies have found expanded access after adopting carve outs (Callahan et al. 1995, Goldman et al. 1998) while others found modest declines in the receipt of appropriate care (Ma and McGuire 1998). One study examining carve outs of pharmacy benefits found that including the benefit in the plan (a "carve in") allowed plans to improve integration of the management of the enrollees' formularies and mix of drugs, resulting in relatively greater use of lower-cost generic drugs and improved care coordination (Joines et al. 2007).

References

Blumenthal, D., and M.B. Buntin. 1998. Carve outs: Definition, experience, and choice among candidate conditions. *The American Journal of Managed Care* 4, special issue: SP45-SP57.

Callahan, J.J., D.S. Shepard, R.H. Beinecke, et al. 1995. Mental health/substance abuse treatment in managed care: The Massachusetts Medicaid experience. *Health Affairs* 14, no. 3: 173-184.

Centers for Medicare & Medicaid Services (CMS), Department of Health and Human Services. Medicaid managed care enrollment report, 1998-2010. https://www.cms.gov/MedicaidDataSourcesGenInfo/04_MdManCrEnrllRep.asp.

Centers for Medicare & Medicaid Services (CMS), Department of Health and Human Services. 2009. National summary of state Medicaid managed care programs. https://www.cms.gov/MedicaidDataSourcesGenInfo/downloads/2009NationalSummaryReport.pdf.

Felt-Lisk, S., R. Dodge, and M. McHugh. 2001. *Trends in health plans serving Medicaid—2000 data update. Report to Kaiser Commission on Medicaid and the Uninsured by Mathematica Policy Research*. November. http://www.kff.org/insurance/loader.cfm?url=/commonspot/security/getfile.cfm&PageID=13885.

Goldman, W., J. McCoulloch, and R. Sturm. 1998. Costs and utilization of mental health services before and after managed care. *Health Affairs* 17, no. 2: 40-52.

Joines, W., J. Menges, and J. Tracey. 2007. *Programmatic assessment of carve-in and carve-out arrangements for Medicaid prescription drugs. Report to the Association for Community Affiliated Plans by The Lewin Group*. http://www.lewin.com/content/publications/AssessmentCarveinCarveOut.pdf.

Ma, C.A., and T. McGuire. 1998. Costs and incentives in a behavioral health carve out. *Health Affairs* 17, no. 2: 53-69.

New York State Department of Health (NY). 2011. *Medicaid redesign initiatives*. Albany, NY: New York State Department of Health. http://www.health.state.ny.us/health_care/managed_care/appextension/mrt_waiver_materials/docs/medicaid_redesign_initiatives.pdf.

Texas Health and Human Services Commission (TX). 2011. *Medicaid managed care proposals*. Austin, TX: Texas Health and Human Services Commission. http://www.hhsc.state.tx.us/medicaid/MMC-Proposals.shtml.

Verdier, J., V. Byrd, and C. Stone. 2009. *Enhanced primary care case management programs in Medicaid: Issues and options for states. Report to Center for Health Care Strategies and Oklahoma Health Care Authority Center*. Washington, DC: Mathematica Policy Research. September. http://www.chcs.org/usr_doc/EPCCM_Full_Report.pdf.

Section C Annex

Medicaid Managed Care Definitions[1]

Managed care entity. A Medicaid managed care organization or primary care case manager (§1932 of the Act).

Comprehensive risk contract. A risk contract that covers inpatient hospital services plus any one of the following services, or at least three of the following services: outpatient hospital, rural health clinic, federally qualified health center, other lab and X-ray, nursing facility, EPSDT, family planning, home health.

Risk contract. A contract under which the managed care contractor assumes risk for the cost of services covered and incurs loss if the cost of furnishing the services exceeds the payments under the contract.

Nonrisk contract. A contract under which the contractor is not at financial risk for changes in utilization or for costs incurred. The contractor may be reimbursed at the end of the contract period on the basis of incurred costs.

Capitation payment. A periodic payment made by a state agency to a contractor on behalf of each enrollee enrolled under a contract for the provision of Medicaid services; payment is made periodically, generally per member per month.

Entities referred to as comprehensive risk-based plans in this Report

- **Managed care organization.** An entity that has or is seeking a comprehensive risk contract.

- **Health insuring organization.** A county-operated entity that covers services through payments to or arrangements with providers, in exchange for capitation payments under a comprehensive risk contract. There are only four HIOs, all in California, as described by the Consolidated Omnibus Budget Reconciliation Act of 1985 (P.L. 99-272).

---

[1] Unless otherwise noted, these terms are defined within 42 CFR 438.2.

Entities referred to as limited-benefit plans in this Report

▶ **Prepaid inpatient health plan (PIHP).** An entity that does not have a comprehensive risk contract; provides, arranges, or otherwise has responsibility for inpatient hospital or institutional services for its enrollees; and is paid on the basis of prepaid capitation payments or other payment arrangement that does not use state plan rates. The most common kind of PIHP is for inpatient mental health services.

▶ **Prepaid ambulatory health plan (PAHP).** An entity that does not have a comprehensive risk contract; provides services other than inpatient hospital or institutional services for its enrollees; and is paid on the basis of prepaid capitation payments or another payment arrangement that does not use state plan rates. Some common PAHPs are for transportation services and oral health services.

Primary Care Case Management (PCCM) Programs

▶ **Primary care case management.** A system under which a primary care case manager (physician, physician group, or entity that employs or arranges with physicians) contracts with a state to furnish case management services, which include location, coordination, and monitoring of primary care. States may also opt to use physician assistants, nurse practitioners, and/or certified nurse midwives.

SECTION

Payment Policy in Medicaid Managed Care

As discussed throughout this Report, there are three primary arrangements through which states typically provide and pay for services in Medicaid managed care: comprehensive risk-based plans, primary care case management (PCCM) programs, and limited-benefit plans. Medicaid managed care payment amounts and methodologies to set rates vary depending on the scope of services and populations covered by these programs as well as whether the plans are at risk for the cost of services.

Medicaid managed care programs, including all comprehensive risk-based plans and many limited-benefit plans, often involve risk-based contracts, which are the primary focus of this section. Under a risk-based contract, the managed care plan assumes financial risk for the cost of covered services and plan administration; the plan could incur a loss if these expenses exceed the payments that the state makes to the plan. Other managed care arrangements may operate under non-risk contracts and therefore are not at risk for a loss based on the cost of services used by enrollees.

States typically pay for risk-based managed care services through fixed periodic (usually monthly) payments for a defined package of benefits. These payments are commonly known as capitation payments; they are typically made on a per member per month (PMPM) basis. Risk-based plans typically negotiate with providers to provide services to their enrollees, either on a fee-for-service (FFS) basis, or through arrangements under which they pay providers (e.g., primary care providers (PCPs)) a fixed periodic amount to provide services. In the case of PCCM programs, providers typically receive a small monthly payment to provide case management services to enrollees in addition to FFS payments for other care rendered.

This section:

- provides an overview of the federal statutes and regulations that govern states' payments to Medicaid managed care plans;

- describes various approaches to managed care payment; and

- explains how states determine capitation rates.

Statutory and Regulatory Overview

Federal statute requires that Medicaid payments be consistent with efficiency, economy, and quality; avoid payment for unnecessary utilization; and are sufficient to enlist enough providers (§1902(a)(30)(A) of the Social Security Act (the Act)). Additionally, the Omnibus Budget Reconciliation Act of 1981 (OBRA 1981, P.L. 97-35) added the requirement that capitation payments to risk-based managed care plans be made on an actuarially sound basis (§1903(m)(2)(A)(iii) of the Act).

Prior to 2002, federal regulations provided little guidance regarding actuarial soundness, limiting capitation payments to an upper payment limit (UPL) equal to the cost of providing the same services in FFS Medicaid to an actuarially equivalent population group (42 CFR 447.361 [repealed]). While the statute required the rates to be actuarially sound, the UPL placed more emphasis on setting a ceiling for rates rather than establishing a floor.

Under the UPL requirement, states used baseline FFS data to compare to expenditures under managed care. However, after several years of providing services through managed care plans for large segments of their Medicaid population, many states were finding it increasingly difficult to make meaningful comparisons to FFS Medicaid since recent FFS data were no longer available

(CMS 2001). In addition the FFS data may not have been useful for comparison purposes. For example, FFS data may have reflected lower levels of preventive screenings and services such as vaccinations than were typical for managed care plans (American Academy of Actuaries 2005).

To address these issues, CMS replaced the UPL requirement in 2002 with regulations codifying the statutory requirement that states' capitation rates under risk contracts be actuarially sound (42 CFR 438.6(c)). The regulations require that state Medicaid managed care rates be developed in accordance with generally accepted actuarial principles and practices, appropriate for the population and services, and certified by qualified actuaries.

The regulations further require that, in setting actuarially sound rates, states must apply the following (or explain why the requirements are not applicable) (42 CFR 438.6(c)(3)):

- base utilization and cost data for the applicable Medicaid population or, if not, adjusted to make the data comparable to the Medicaid population;

- adjustments to smooth data and to account for factors such as medical trend inflation, incomplete data, and utilization;

- rates specific to eligibility category, age, gender, locality/region, and diagnosis or health status (if used); and

- other mechanisms and assumptions that are appropriate for individuals with chronic illness, disability, ongoing health care needs, or catastrophic claims, using risk adjustment, risk sharing, or other appropriate cost-neutral methods.

These requirements apply to comprehensive risk-based Medicaid managed care plans as well as risk-based limited-benefit plans, such as those providing only oral or behavioral health benefits.

States must demonstrate their compliance with the actuarial soundness requirements to CMS by documenting their rate-setting methodology and the base utilization data used to set rates. CMS staff use a checklist to verify states' compliance with these requirements. The checklist includes statutory and regulatory citations for specific requirements, descriptions of methods for complying with requirements, and a place for CMS staff to indicate whether or not requirements have been met. Sections covered by the checklist include:

- general requirements (e.g., actuarial certification, contracting process);
- base year utilization and cost data;
- adjustments to the base year data;
- rate category groupings (e.g., age, gender, locality);
- data smoothing, special populations, and catastrophic claims;
- stop-loss, reinsurance, or risk-sharing arrangements; and
- incentive arrangements.

A recent study by the Government Accountability Office (GAO) found that CMS' oversight of states' compliance with actuarial soundness requirements and data quality for rate setting could be improved (GAO 2010). The GAO noted that CMS used elements of the checklist inconsistently and that the depth of CMS reviews varied. CMS concurred with the report's findings and indicated that steps were already being taken to address them, including the development of new protocols, a revised checklist, and formal sub-regulatory guidance, as well as expanded data collection and quality reviews.

The American Academy of Actuaries (the Academy) is also working to improve rate setting in Medicaid managed care programs. Although no actuarial standard of practice (ASOP) applies specifically to Medicaid managed care rate setting, the Academy published a practice note in 2005 that defined actuarial soundness for Medicaid. Under this definition rates are actuarially sound if they "provide for all reasonable, appropriate, and attainable costs" that are incurred by plans (American Academy of Actuaries 2005). The Academy has also convened a task force to begin developing an ASOP for Medicaid managed care rate setting.

Non-risk-based managed care plans are typically paid a fixed administrative fee, rather than a capitation payment. These payments must be no more than what the state would have paid for services under traditional FFS plus the net savings of administrative costs the Medicaid agency achieves by contracting with the plan (42 CFR 447.362). Federal matching payments for administrative fees are limited to the federal matching rate for administrative expenses (typically 50 percent). However, the amount states pay for medical assistance under a non-risk contract is subject to the state's federal medical assistance percentage (FMAP).

Approaches to Managed Care Plan Payment

The approaches that states use for determining capitation payments to comprehensive risk-based plans depend on the methods that they use to contract with these plans. In general the following approaches are used to establish rates:

- **Administered pricing.** With administered pricing, capitation payments are determined by the state; plans determine whether or not they wish to apply for participation in the program.

▶ **Competitive bidding.** In this approach, states typically issue a request for proposals (RFP) and then select managed care plans based on an evaluation of their proposed rates and services.

States may also use hybrid approaches, such as setting a range of rates and then asking plans to bid competitively within that range, or negotiating with plans based on the administered pricing or their competitive bids.

Information on state contracting approaches is somewhat dated, with the most recent surveys of states occurring in 2001 and 2006. Based on the 2001 survey, administered pricing was the most common, used by 19 of the 36 states that responded. Ten states reported using competitive bidding, and seven states indicated that they negotiated with plans individually (Holahan and Suzuki 2003). In the 2001 survey, several states that had reported using competitive bidding in a 1998 survey had switched by 2001 to administered pricing. That trend continued in 2006, when a survey of states and plans found that only five of 21 responding states used competitive bidding (Catterall et al. 2006).

Administered pricing allows states to set rates at the lower end of an actuarially sound range, rather than having to accept a competitive bid potentially at the higher end of the range. States may use administered pricing, for example, when faced with budgetary limitations.

When considering whether to participate in Medicaid managed care, plans may also consider factors other than payment rates. For example, some states use auto-assignment to assign a portion of enrollees to participating plans. This could encourage plans to participate even at a potentially lower payment rate because auto-assignment assures that these plans are able to enroll a portion of those individuals that do not select a plan. Both statute (§1932(a)(3) of the Act) and regulations

(42 CFR 438.52) generally require that enrollees be given a choice of managed care plans (there is an exception for rural area residents). However, states may auto-assign individuals that do not make a choice within specified time limits.

Rate Setting

In determining capitation rates, states and plans use data and adjustment factors to predict enrollees' use of health care services and the expected cost of these services. Setting rates typically involves consideration of a number of factors, including:

▶ baseline data;

▶ expected trends;

▶ state fiscal conditions;

▶ services that are carved out of managed care;

▶ payments in addition to the base capitation rate; and

▶ incentives.

Baseline data. Depending on the type of contracting method that a state chooses, states or plans typically set rates based on either FFS or managed care services and utilization data (known as encounter data) if available, or both. In general, when a state first establishes a managed care program, recent FFS utilization and spending data are available to estimate rates.

Over time, as more enrollees move into managed care and these programs become more established, current FFS claims are less available and less reliable as a benchmark for establishing capitation rates. Instead many states and plans have come to rely more on encounter data or aggregate spending by service type, as well as financial reports submitted by the plans, to project utilization and spending in the coming year. Depending on data availability and quality, states and plans may prefer to use encounter and financial data to reflect more precisely the health status of and spending for individuals enrolled in managed care plans. States may also use a combination of FFS, encounter, and financial data.

Expected trends. States and plans establish capitation rates by trending baseline spending and utilization data (either FFS or encounter data) forward to establish an expected per member per month amount. Rates incorporate expected costs to administer the plan (including care management activities not routinely conducted under FFS) and may also explicitly allow for some profit margin for the plan.

Some states also adjust rates to account for efficiency factors. Efficiency factors adjust the capitation payment for services that managed care plans are expected to manage, thus creating an incentive to reduce the use of these services over time. Payment rates may be adjusted to account for better management of services, including reductions in emergency department (ED) services, unnecessary inpatient admissions, or the use of brand name drugs when a generic substitute is available.

State fiscal conditions. While rates are required to be actuarially sound regardless of state budget pressures, states have proposed reductions in managed care payments when faced with budget limitations. For example, states may set managed care rates assuming reductions in profit margins, marketing costs, and other factors. In addition to the decisions that states make directly about managed care rates, decisions about FFS provider payment rates can also have an indirect effect on managed care rates. For example, FFS rate reductions could result in a reduction in managed care payments in a state that bases managed care rates on FFS rates.

Carve outs. Payments to plans take into account spending for any carve outs or benefits that are excluded from the managed care program (e.g., behavioral health, transportation, oral health). Medicaid managed care enrollees may still be able to access these services through FFS Medicaid or through a limited-benefit plan that is contracted to provide these services.

Additional Payments. In addition to rate adjustments for carve outs, some states make additional payments for certain services to managed care plans, commonly known as "kick payments." These payments (often one-time, fixed payments) allow plans to cover particular services without assuming the financial risk for their use. The costs for these services are then excluded from the capitation rate setting process. Maternity kick payments are commonly made to Medicaid managed care plans as Medicaid is a major payer for these services. These kick payments minimize the financial risk to plans of women enrolling in plans late in their pregnancies. Most of the states surveyed in 2001 reported making direct payments to plans for the expected cost of maternity services (Holahan and Suzuki 2003). In some states these payments are increased for low birth weight infants. Some states also make kick payments for transplant services, rather than include the cost of these services in capitation rates.

Incentives. Some states also include incentive payments in their rate setting process. For example, the New York State Medicaid program may make incentive payments of up to 3 percent of per member per month payments to plans with high ratings on performance measures. Participating plans that earn the quality bonus may also be rewarded for high performance by receiving the auto-assignment of enrollees who did not select a plan upon enrollment (New York State Department of Health 2007).

Risk Adjustment

As previously mentioned, federal regulations (42 CFR 438.6(c)(3)) require states to account for the following factors (or explain why they are not applicable): eligibility category, age, gender, locality/region, and diagnosis or health status in their capitation rates and to apply techniques such as risk sharing and risk adjustment to account for individuals with higher health care costs. Traditionally states have adjusted plan payment rates for demographic factors such as those above, for example, by paying higher rates for older enrollees. Over time, however, demographic factors alone have been shown to be relatively weak predictors of spending and service use, especially compared to factors based on diagnosis and health care history (Winkelman and Damler 2008). A growing number of states have begun to adjust rates based on enrollee health status to reflect a plan's mix of enrollees and their expected care needs and expenditures.

Risk adjustment helps assure that health plans receive payment sufficient to cover the costs of delivering and arranging care efficiently without compromising quality and access. Ultimately, the accuracy of risk adjustment can affect plans' willingness to participate in Medicaid managed care, particularly for more complex populations (e.g., those dually eligible for both Medicaid and Medicare (dual eligibles) or those with disabilities and/or mental health conditions). These methodologies can also protect against creating unintended incentives for adverse selection or "cherry picking" healthier enrollees within some of these complex populations.

Risk adjustment uses a variety of factors including both demographics and health status to refine rates and to pay more for individuals who are likely to have higher health care costs. Some risk adjustment methodologies include health status information gathered from medical claims or encounter data

to develop risk-based weights for a variety of different enrollees. Others use pharmacy data to risk adjust rates. Some of the methodologies used by states for risk adjustment include the Chronic Illness and Disability Payment System (CDPS), Adjusted Clinical Groups (ACG), Diagnostic Cost Groups (DxCG), MedicaidRx, and a Clinical Risk Groups pharmacy add on (CRxG).

While risk adjustment is a common practice throughout the private insurance markets and Medicare, there may be particular factors that need to be taken into account in developing accurate risk adjustment mechanisms for Medicaid. For example, Medicaid enrollees have a higher incidence of behavioral health issues than is prevalent in the general population. Regardless of whether behavioral health services are included within Medicaid managed care plan benefits, including the use of behavioral health services in the risk adjustment methodology may be helpful because mental health conditions can exacerbate other medical conditions (Winkelman and Damler 2008).

In the case of dual eligibles, because acute care services are primarily paid for by Medicare, risk adjustment techniques are specifically needed to estimate the use and costs of long-term services and supports in Medicaid. Wisconsin, for example, uses information on enrollees' activities of daily living, other characteristics such as level of care, and expenditures to develop payment adjustments (Kronick and Llanos 2008).

Risk Sharing

In some cases states have incorporated contract provisions in which the state shares some of the risk borne by managed care plans. These may include risk corridors, stop-loss or reinsurance provisions, and other similar arrangements.

BOX D-1. Challenges in Comparing Medicaid Managed Care Rates

It is difficult to compare Medicaid managed care rates across states and the results of such comparisons may not be informative regarding the appropriateness of rates. Studies have shown more than a two-fold variation in managed care rates across states (Holahan and Suzuki 2003); however, this does not necessarily mean that individual states are overpaying or underpaying for managed care services. Reasons for variation in managed care rates include the following:

- State programs include different benefit packages; decisions to include or exclude benefits such as prescription drugs and behavioral health services have a significant impact on rates.
- Programs that cover only lower-cost enrollees such as mothers and children have much lower rates than those that include older and/or disabled populations.
- In some states, maternity costs are included in the capitation rate while in others these costs are paid through "kick payments".
- Medical costs vary across states and affect the rates that plans are able to negotiate with providers.
- Other market dynamics, such as the number of practitioners competing for business, affect the rates at which plans are able to contract with providers.

As a result of these and other factors, Medicaid managed care rates can vary significantly without necessarily resulting in variations in actuarial soundness. However, the numerous factors that result in variation in rates also limit state and federal regulators' ability to evaluate the suitability of rates or to isolate the impact of individual cost drivers.

Risk corridors. In a risk corridor arrangement, plans may be responsible for absorbing only a certain percentage of losses if aggregate spending for services exceeds the plan's capitation payments. The state will reimburse the plan for the remainder of the losses. If, on the other hand, payments for services are less than the amount paid by the state in capitation payments, plans are able to retain the savings up to a certain percentage, beyond which they are required to return a portion of the savings to the state. Because risk-sharing techniques are required by federal regulation to be computed on an actuarially sound basis, there are federal limits on the amount of savings that plans can retain (42 CFR 438.6(c)(5)).

Stop-loss/Reinsurance. Some contracts also contain "stop-loss" or "reinsurance" provisions that protect plans from losses beyond predetermined thresholds on an individual basis

(e.g., $50,000 in payments for a single enrollee). Beyond the specified threshold, states will assume some or all of the enrollee's cost of care. When states use such thresholds, capitation rates are adjusted to account for the reduced risk that the plans bear. Managed care plans may also choose to purchase reinsurance in the private market. As an alternative to stop-loss, states may keep enrollees with high-cost health conditions (e.g., hemophilia, HIV/AIDS) out of managed care programs to lower the risk borne by plans.

No up-to-date source of comprehensive information currently exists regarding the payment approaches, risk adjustment, incentives, and other arrangements used by states in contracting with comprehensive risk-based plans for Medicaid services. As part of the Commission's work to better define the Medicaid payment landscape, we plan to work to understand these methods.

PCCM Payment

Under PCCM programs, PCPs are typically paid a monthly amount (e.g., $3 per enrollee) to coordinate services and to influence the appropriate use of specialists and hospital services. These providers are still paid on a FFS basis for the medical services that they provide. Under a PCCM program, the state continues to bear the financial risk for the cost of services provided to enrollees, a key distinction between PCCM programs and risk-based plans.

Increasingly, states have been adopting a type of PCCM program generally referred to as "enhanced PCCM". In these programs states may provide incentive payments to promote quality, increased care coordination, and management of complex chronic conditions. For example, Oklahoma, Pennsylvania, and Indiana all use predictive modeling software to identify enrollees most likely to benefit from enhanced care coordination. Each of these states then seeks to coordinate care for a range of these enrollees' health needs, rather than focusing on individual conditions (Verdier et al. 2009).

BOX D-2. Implications of Upper Payment Limit Payments for Medicaid Managed Care

As discussed in the Commission's March 2011 Report, some states make supplemental payments to hospital and other institutional providers under FFS arrangements, above what they pay for individual services. States make these payments under the federal Upper Payment Limit (UPL) regulation (42 CFR 447) and claim federal matching dollars. These UPL supplemental payments may be a large revenue source for hospitals and other institutional providers, especially safety-net providers. These payments have implications for state expansion of Medicaid managed care. Since the UPL is based on only FFS days in a hospital or institutional setting, transitioning populations from FFS to managed care would mean fewer FFS days and lower UPL supplemental payments.

States have had to consider this potential reduction in supplemental payments and federal matching funds as they look to expand managed care to additional populations and services (McKethan and Menges 2006). According to federal requirements (42 CFR 438.60), services covered by Medicaid managed care plans must be considered "paid in full" through the capitation payment to the managed care plan. Thus, supplemental payments are not permitted within risk-based managed care.

If the shift in inpatient days from FFS to managed care is large enough, the loss of federal matching dollars for UPL payments can offset savings that may be realized through managed care, resulting in a net loss to states and a significant reduction in total payments to hospitals. This issue may be greater for more complex populations that use more days in an institutional setting, such as SSI enrollees. Because the UPL is based on the number of days of care, moving higher-use populations to managed care has a larger impact on UPL payments. On the other hand, enrolling populations like children and parents who typically use fewer inpatient days has less of an impact on supplemental payment amounts and has not been a major factor in enrolling these populations in managed care.

A few states have delayed implementation or expansion of Medicaid managed care because of the potential loss in federal matching dollars for supplemental payments, and in some cases have applied for Section 1115 waiver authority to address this issue. In 2005, Florida was granted a waiver that preserved some amount of their hospital supplemental payments. In Texas, the state carved out inpatient care from the Star Plus program to preserve supplemental payments and is developing a Section 1115 waiver to address this issue as part of a managed care expansion.

In addition to paying individual providers for services, some states have contracted with vendors to provide additional care management or disease management activities. Some states have also placed a portion of disease management payments at risk, based on the level of savings that vendors are able to achieve. Examples include Pennsylvania's Access Plus program and Texas' Medicaid Wellness Program.

A number of PCCM programs include HEDIS-based clinical quality measurement of PCPs and also offer performance-based incentive payments. Oklahoma includes a performance-based payment component for providers that meet quality targets in areas including immunizations, breast and cervical cancer screenings, generic drug prescribing, ED use, and inpatient admissions (OKHCA 2011). Pennsylvania's pay-for-performance program includes bonus payments to providers for supporting program participation as well as clinical measures in a variety of areas including chronic disease management, women's health, and pediatric health (APS Healthcare 2010). In Indiana, a portion of care management organization payments is withheld and paid out based on measures related to ED utilization, preventive care, and chronic disease management. A portion of these payments must be reinvested as incentive payments to providers and members (Verdier et al. 2009).

Recent Payment Provisions

The Patient Protection and Affordable Care Act (PPACA, P.L. 111-148) as amended by the Health Care and Education Reconciliation Act (P.L. 111-152) includes several provisions that will affect Medicaid managed care payment. One provision requires states to pay 100 percent of the Medicare payment amount for primary care services provided by family medicine, general internal medicine, or pediatric medicine physicians participating in Medicaid during calendar years 2013 and 2014. Medicaid managed care plans must also make payments to physicians consistent with these new minimum payment amounts.

CMS also recently published a final rule implementing the PPACA requirement that states reduce or prohibit payments to providers for services that result from certain preventable health care acquired illnesses or injuries. The new rule requires states to include these payment restrictions in their managed care contracts (CMS 2011).

PPACA also includes provisions to encourage the use of health care service delivery models such as health homes and accountable care organizations (ACOs). The adoption of such models by states and their managed care plans may require modifications to existing payment approaches and, in some cases, the development of new approaches. The Commission will continue to examine these and other aspects of managed care payment moving forward.

References

American Academy of Actuaries, Medicaid Rate Certification Work Group. 2005. *Actuarial certification of rates for Medicaid managed care programs.* Washington, DC: American Academy of Actuaries. http://www.actuary.org/pdf/practnotes/health_medicaid_05.pdf.

APS Healthcare. 2010. Pay for performance. http://www.accessplus.org/providers/providers-programs/providers-programs-pay_per_performance.aspx.

Catterall, G., L. Chimento, R. Sethi, and B. Maughan. 2006. *Rate setting and actuarial soundness in Medicaid managed care. Report to the Association for Community Affiliated Plans and Medicaid Health Plans of America by the Lewin Group.* January 23. http://www.mhpa.org/pdf/misc/ACAP_MHPOAreport.pdf.

Centers for Medicare & Medicaid Services (CMS), Department of Health and Human Services. 2011. Medicaid program: Payment adjustment for provider-preventable conditions including health care-acquired conditions. Final rule. *Federal Register* 76, no. 108 (June 6): 32816-32838.

Centers for Medicare & Medicaid Services (CMS), Department of Health and Human Services. 2001. Medicaid program; Medicaid managed care. Proposed rule. *Federal Register* 66, no. 161 (August 20): 43614-43677.

Government Accountability Office (GAO). 2010. *Medicaid managed care: CMS's oversight of states' rate setting needs improvement.* Washington, DC: GAO. http://www.gao.gov/new.items/d10810.pdf.

Holahan, J., and S. Suzuki. 2003. Medicaid managed care payment methods and capitation rates in 2001. *Health Affairs* 22, no.1: 204-218.

Kronick, R., and K. Llanos. 2008. *Rate-setting for Medicaid managed long-term supports and services: Best practices and recommendations for states. Report to the Robert Wood Johnson Foundation by the Center for Health Care Strategies (CHCS).* March. http://www.chcs.org/usr_doc/Rate_Setting_for_Medicaid_MLTS.pdf.

McKethan, A., and J. Menges. 2006. *Medicaid upper payment limit policies: Overcoming a barrier to managed care expansion. Report to Medicaid Health Plans of America by the Lewin Group.* November 13. http://www.lewin.com/content/publications/UPL.pdf.

New York State Department of Health, Office of Health Insurance Programs. 2007. *Quality strategy for the New York state Medicaid managed care program.* http://www.health.state.ny.us/health_care/managed_care/docs/quality_strategy.pdf.

Oklahoma Health Care Authority (OKHCA). 2011. SoonerExcel. Oklahoma City: Oklahoma Health Care Authority website. http://www.okhca.org/providers.aspx?id=9426&menu=74&parts=8482_10165.

Verdier, J., V. Byrd, and C. Stone. 2009. *Enhanced primary care case management programs in Medicaid: Issues and options for states. Report to Center for Health Care Strategies and Oklahoma Health Care Authority Center by Mathematica Policy Research.* September. http://www.chcs.org/usr_doc/EPCCM_Full_Report.pdf.

Winkelman, R., and R. Damler. 2008. Risk adjustment in state Medicaid programs. *Health Watch* 57: 14-34. http://www.soa.org/library/newsletters/health-watch-newsletter/2008/january/hsn-2008-iss57-damler-winkelman.pdf.

SECTION

Access and Quality in Managed Care

Contracting with managed care plans creates the potential for some states to improve access to appropriate services, better coordinate care for Medicaid enrollees, and measure performance with regard to quality. Medicaid managed care links enrollees with a primary care provider (PCP) or case manager and, in doing so, offers opportunities for improved continuity and care coordination. Capitated payment and other managed care features can also be designed to emphasize prevention and early detection of health conditions. However, poorly designed or implemented Medicaid managed care programs can also create issues for states that may lead to poor enrollee health outcomes. In addition, there may be considerations for managed care in addressing the needs of certain populations or geographic areas.

Standards, reporting, and enforcement of Medicaid managed care contract requirements vary considerably across states. This variation among states creates challenges for comparing and assessing access and quality. The ability to synthesize research across states is also constrained because individual studies typically provide national estimates or focus only on one or a few states and vary considerably in the measures used, their comprehensiveness, and their research quality; many studies in this area are also dated. Current national surveys have limitations, such as the absence of sufficient state-level sample sizes, the time lag in gathering and reporting survey data, the lack of information on whether or not individuals are enrolled in managed care, and the limited range of access measures that can be self-reported.

This section:

» reviews how comprehensive risk-based Medicaid managed care relates to each dimension of access defined in the Commission's March 2011 Report to the Congress (MACPAC 2011);

» describes quality measurement and improvement activities most commonly used by states; and identifies the importance of data and updated analyses to assess access and quality in Medicaid managed care.

Monitoring Access in Comprehensive Risk-based Managed Care

The Commission's initial access framework was developed in order to guide our future work on access to care and services for Medicaid and CHIP enrollees. Drawing upon over 30 years of research on defining and measuring access to care, the framework provides an approach that considers the complex characteristics and health needs of the Medicaid and CHIP populations, as well as program variability across states. We expect our access framework to evolve to address new health care practice patterns, changing program needs, and new areas of focus.

The Commission's initial framework for monitoring access to care focuses on three main elements: enrollees and their unique characteristics, provider availability, and appropriate utilization:

- **Enrollees.** Medicaid and CHIP enrollees have unique characteristics to be accounted for in monitoring access to care.

- **Availability.** Provider availability for Medicaid and CHIP enrollees affects access and is influenced by provider supply and provider participation.

- **Utilization.** An assessment of access to care should focus on whether appropriate and available services are used, the affordability of services, the enrollee's ability to navigate the health care system, and the enrollee's experiences with the health care system.

These three components will serve as the basis for the Commission to evaluate access, including the appropriateness of services and settings, efficiency, economy, and quality of care, and impact on health outcomes.

Enrollees

Medicaid enrollees have unique health care needs and characteristics to be accounted for in monitoring access to care, including demographic characteristics and the ways in which they qualify for coverage. Section B of this Report discusses the characteristics of the various eligibility groups and potential challenges related to their enrollment in managed care. Issues particularly salient to access to care for Medicaid enrollees include:

- frequent turnover in eligibility;

- complex, chronic medical needs that may benefit from care coordination, care management, and continuity of care;

- provider networks that include adequate numbers of PCPs and specialists who treat health issues such as behavioral health needs that are more common in the Medicaid population; and

- coordination with Medicare on care and benefits for those dually eligible for Medicaid and Medicare.

These issues may have implications for how Medicaid enrollees experience access to care in managed care settings.

Frequent turnover in eligibility may mean that enrollees have intermittent access to the same providers during the year. If individuals re-enroll, there is a chance they could be enrolled in different plans with different provider networks and face challenges in maintaining continuity of care (March 2011 MACStats Table 1).

Complex medical needs lead many Medicaid enrollees to require more provider visits during the year than are typically used by individuals not enrolled in Medicaid (MACStats Tables 3C, 4C, 5C). Thus, Medicaid managed care provider networks may need to include a larger and more specialized set of providers to facilitate adequate access. This may be particularly true as states increasingly move to enroll children with special health care needs and adults with disabilities into managed care plans.

Specialty care needs may also differ for the Medicaid population compared to the privately insured population. For example, child and adult Medicaid/CHIP enrollees are more likely than the privately insured to have certain health conditions that may require specialty care (MACStats Tables 3B, 4B).

Dual eligibility for Medicare and Medicaid can create particular challenges for Medicaid managed care enrollees. Dual eligibles may have access to a very different set of providers for their Medicare-covered benefits compared to the benefits covered by their Medicaid managed care plan. Nearly all providers participate in fee-for-service (FFS) Medicare; if a dual eligible is instead enrolled in a Medicare Advantage (MA) plan, that plan may have a network of providers that is different from the enrollee's Medicaid managed care network of providers. States are currently exploring ways to improve coordination of the two programs, as described in Section B of this Report.

Availability of Providers

For all Medicaid enrollees, provider availability is influenced by provider supply in their geographic area and the share of those providers that agree to participate in Medicaid. Concerns about both provider supply and provider participation affect both traditional FFS Medicaid and Medicaid managed care programs. Provider participation may vary because health providers voluntarily choose whether or not to participate in these programs.[1] Managed care offers states additional mechanisms for assessing and influencing the adequacy of provider participation in Medicaid. Through their contracts with participating managed care plans, states can require compliance with standards for network adequacy.

One of the most detailed studies of provider networks in Medicaid and CHIP health plans comes from a 2001 survey of health plans in 11 states with the largest plan enrollment (Gold et al. 2003). At that time, most plans said that they experienced few problems developing and maintaining their provider networks, but reported more problems with specialist contracting than with PCPs, with particular issues in certain specialties (e.g., pediatric subspecialties).

As a preliminary step to understanding the current landscape of monitoring access across states and examining access to care in Medicaid, the Commission requested information from state Medicaid directors in the 50 states and the District of Columbia from November 2010 through April 2011. The questionnaire was designed to compile timely information on how states monitor and identify potential provider supply problems. Findings from the questionnaire are presented in the Annex to this Section.

---

[1] While state legislatures could require health professionals to participate in Medicaid or CHIP as a condition of licensure or gaining other valued commodities, opposition to such policies makes enactment difficult (Gold and Aizer 2000).

Appropriate Utilization

Because Medicaid coverage does not guarantee access to services and may not ensure appropriate use of services, an analysis of utilization for the purpose of assessing access to care needs to focus on:

▸ whether or not appropriate, available services are obtained;

▸ the affordability of services;

▸ the enrollee's ability to navigate the health care system; and

▸ the enrollee's experiences with the health care system.

In an effort to improve outcomes and reduce costs, managed care programs aim to better manage the use of health care services. In FFS Medicaid, enrollees may seek care from any participating provider. Comprehensive risk-based plans often have specific rules regarding appropriate use of services. In both comprehensive risk-based plans and primary care case management (PCCM) programs, enrollees may be required to select a PCP or obtain prior authorization or approval to receive certain tests or visits to specialists unless an emergency situation exists.[2]

Methods for coordinating care and assuring receipt of appropriate services may be clearly delineated in comprehensive risk-based managed care. State contracts may emphasize the need for plans to place a greater focus on enrollees and their health needs, giving plans responsibility for arranging, providing, and overseeing the care of their members consistent with the specified benefit package and medical necessity. Building on the FFS structure, PCCM programs incorporate managed care features such as care management, often using PCPs to perform these activities on behalf of the enrollees.

States require participating comprehensive risk-based plans to ensure that each enrollee has a PCP and that PCP assignments, when necessary, are based on factors such as proximity to an enrollee's home, primary language spoken, and prior PCP relationship. Plans may be required to provide a designated case manager for some individuals with chronic or complex medical conditions who require additional assistance obtaining services. Plans may also be required to establish disease management programs to provide education and clinical guidance to enrollees with specific medical conditions such as asthma or diabetes. Contracts may also specify staffing requirements (e.g., clinically relevant experience, staffing ratios) for individuals coordinating care and providing case management and disease management services.

Monitoring Quality of Care in Comprehensive Risk-based Managed Care

Quality measurement, monitoring, and improvement have received increasing attention in Medicaid. Such interest has been facilitated by increasingly sophisticated and prevalent information technology tools for data collection and analysis, as well as the development of a range of measures for almost all aspects of health care delivery and outcomes (Smith et al. 2010). Payers have exhibited a marked interest in using these population-based measures to gauge the value and quality of the services they purchase (Rosenbaum et al. 2003).

Medicaid programs are using information from managed care plans to set standards, structure payment, measure performance, and provide comparison reports to consumers. To help Medicaid enrollees choose a managed care plan,

---

[2] States may also use utilization management tools such as prior authorization in their FFS programs.

BOX E-1.   Updated Analyses Would Support Program Evaluation

Available evidence on the overall impact of comprehensive risk-based managed care on utilization, receipt of appropriate services, and quality of care in Medicaid is mixed, reflecting differences across states, markets, services, and metrics used for comparison. The studies and data used are generally dated, making it difficult to draw comparisons to state Medicaid managed care programs today. Many study findings may not be applicable to experience today, particularly as states have gained experience with managed care and have become more adept at using the managed care contract as a tool for achieving certain program outcomes. Overall, there is a significant gap in research that does not allow for comparisons of performance among state Medicaid managed care programs in order to determine which techniques are effective (or ineffective) for monitoring the quality, economy, and costs of care. We present examples of available studies for context, but recognize more work is needed in this area.[3]

---

states are also increasingly publishing information on managed care plan performance on websites, in reports, or in the form of report cards. In FY 2010, 41 states indicated that they publicly report health plan performance information (Smith et al. 2010).

States must meet certain requirements established by the Balanced Budget Act of 1997 (P.L. 105-33) and subsequent regulations for monitoring quality of care, but have a fair amount of flexibility in what they report to the federal government (CMS 2002). For example, under 42 CFR 438.240(b), comprehensive risk-based plans must have an ongoing quality assessment and performance improvement program. These requirements are discussed in more detail in Section F of this Report.

States make plans accountable for providing quality care by incorporating quality requirements in their Medicaid managed care contracts. Commonly used

tools for monitoring quality in Medicaid managed care include:

- External quality review organizations (EQROs);
- Healthcare Effectiveness Data and Information Set (HEDIS);[4]
- Consumer Assessment of Healthcare Providers and Systems (CAHPS);[5]
- accreditation; and
- pay for performance.

EQROs

States must provide for an external, independent review of their managed care plans conducted by an EQRO. States must contract with an independent entity, an EQRO, to conduct the review. Comprehensive risk-based plans must have an external quality review (EQR) performed on the quality, timeliness, and access to services they provide (42 CFR 438.310). The external review

---

[3] While some of these studies have been published recently, they are generally based on data as old as the mid-1990s. Examples of available research on access include: Sparer 2008, Bella et al. 2006, CHCF 2004, Chang et al. 2003, Brown et al. 2001, Long and Coughlin 2001, Mitchell et al. 2001, Gold 1999, Lillie-Blanton and Lyons 1998, and McCall and Winter 1997. Examples of research on quality include: GAO 2009, Bollinger et al. 2007, Landon and Epstein 1999, Fontanella et al. 2006, and Aizer et al. 2007.

[4] HEDIS is a registered trademark of the National Committee for Quality Assurance (NCQA).

[5] CAHPS is a registered trademark of the Agency for Healthcare Research and Quality, which oversees the survey.

must include an assessment of the plan's strengths and weaknesses with respect to quality, timeliness, and access to services; recommendations for improving quality of services; and an assessment of how well the plan addressed recommendations from the previous review (42 CFR 438.364). Because federal requirements give states flexibility on what types of services should be reviewed, results are difficult to compare across states. For example, one state might focus on quality of oral health services provided and another on behavioral health services. Results can, however, be used to address performance improvements with managed care plans.

HEDIS

The National Committee for Quality Assurance (NCQA) has created a set of state-level quality, access, and effectiveness-of-care measures for selected conditions known as HEDIS. Many states require their participating plans to collect and report data on these HEDIS measures. Table E-1 includes a sample of select measures from NCQA's *The State of Health Care Quality 2010 Report*, which compares national averages for enrollees in Medicaid managed plans, individuals

with commercial coverage enrolled in a health maintenance organization (HMO), and enrollees in MA HMOs. Scores on all of these measures are lower for Medicaid managed care enrollees than for individuals in other types of plans. For example, the rate of high blood pressure control for Medicaid enrollees is lower than the rates for MA enrollees and for individuals with commercial insurance (55 percent compared to 60 and 64 percent, respectively). However, important differences between the commercial, Medicare, and Medicaid populations such as health status and income may affect the results. In addition, data are only reported for individuals who are continuously enrolled for 12 months, so they may not be representative of the entire Medicaid managed care population. Therefore, comparisons among the populations need to be viewed with caution.

CAHPS

CAHPS is a set of beneficiary surveys designed for children and adults that covers a range of topics, including access to care and use of services, wait times, appointment scheduling, access to specialty care, and satisfaction with providers. For Medicaid programs, CAHPS is an important quality

TABLE E-1. Select HEDIS Effectiveness of Care Measures (National HMO Means, 2009)

Measure	Commercial	Medicare	Medicaid
Use of appropriate medications for people with asthma	92.7%	N/A	88.6%
Prenatal and postpartum care: Timeliness of prenatal care	93.1	N/A	83.4
Controlling high blood pressure	64.1	59.8%	55.3
Weight assessment and counseling for nutrition and physical activity in children and adolescents: Counseling for physical activity	36.5	N/A	32.5

Note: Comparisons among the populations need to be viewed with caution because important differences between the commercial, Medicare, and Medicaid populations may affect the results (i.e., health status, income, and benefit designs of the different programs).
Source: NCQA 2010a

improvement tool used by states and managed care plans to measure performance, determine where to focus improvement efforts, and track improvements over time. Some state Medicaid agencies use CAHPS and similar measures to gauge member satisfaction with Medicaid managed care arrangements. Data from the 2010 CAHPS survey show that enrollees in Medicaid managed care plans gave their health plan a higher overall rating compared to privately insured or Medicare patients (NCQA 2010a). Figure E-1 shows which states require HEDIS and CAHPS measures for Medicaid and for other lines of business.

Accreditation

States may require that managed care plans receive accreditation from an approved accrediting body as a condition of participation in Medicaid. To receive accreditation, plans must meet a set of standards that align with federal requirements for Medicaid managed care. There are several accreditation organizations that states may use in their accreditation processes. For example, NCQA is an accreditation organization that evaluates plans by product line or product (e.g., Medicaid, Medicare, commercial), and plans can receive an accreditation status of Excellent, Commendable, Accredited, Provisional, or Denied. According to NCQA, 25

FIGURE E-1.   Required HEDIS and CAHPS Measures by State, 2010

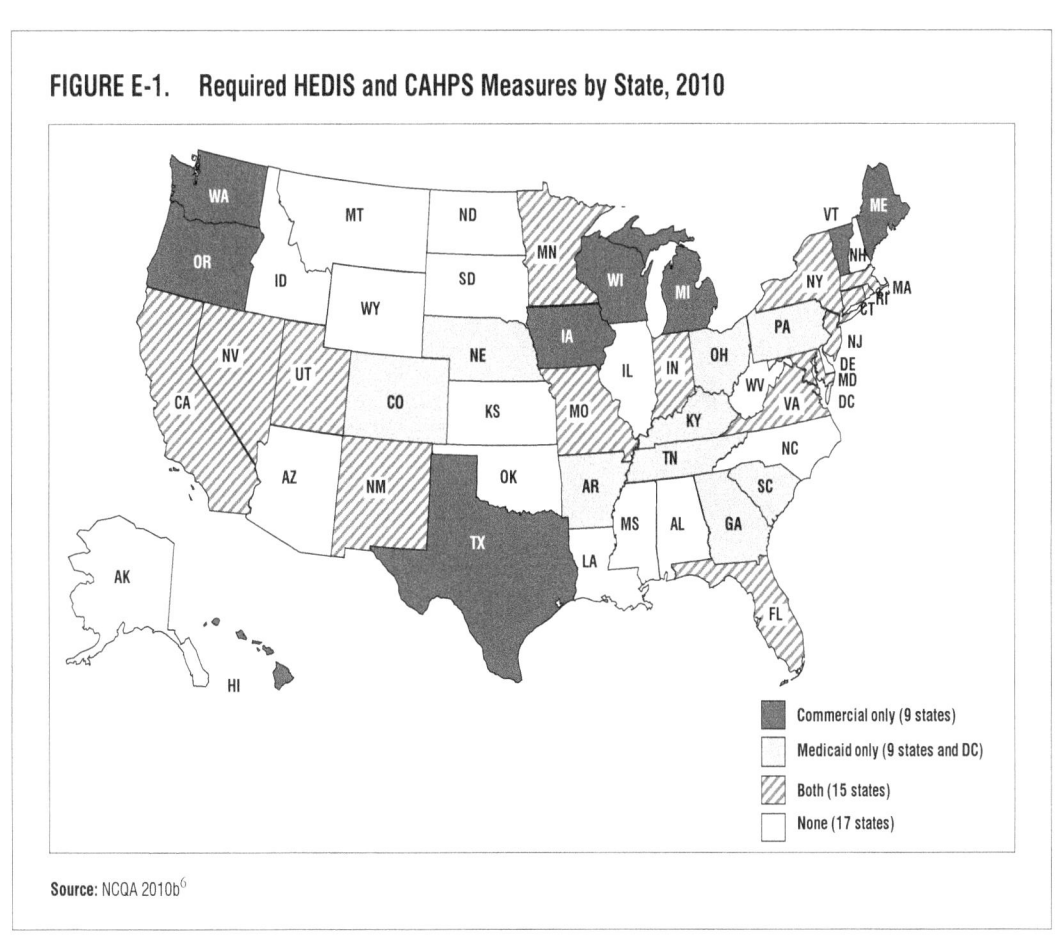

Commercial only (9 states)
Medicaid only (9 states and DC)
Both (15 states)
None (17 states)

Source: NCQA 2010b[6]

---

[6] Some states may only collect HEDIS and CAHPS data for commercial purposes only, particularly if the state has no risk-based managed care.

states recognize or require NCQA accreditation for their Medicaid managed care plans. States requiring NCQA accreditation may use this process to scale back their own state quality monitoring activities (NCQA 2010b). Another accreditation organization, URAC (formerly known as the Utilization Review Accreditation Commission), is also recognized and used by several states for monitoring quality in their Medicaid managed care plans (URAC 2009).

Pay for Performance Incentives

As an increasing number of Medicaid enrollees are in some form of managed care, states have looked for ways to incent plans to provide high quality, accessible, and cost-effective services. In 2010, 34 states reported having "pay for performance" policies and performance-based payment methodologies for plans, including financial incentives (e.g., bonus payments for exceeding performance benchmarks) and nonfinancial incentives (e.g., auto-assignment of Medicaid members into higher performing plans) (Smith et al. 2010).

Plans often routinely report data that states can incorporate into a pay for performance system; most plans have more staff capacity to participate in such a system than individual providers do (Kuhmerker and Hartman 2007). However, there has been little research on the extent to which these pay for performance strategies are associated with improved quality outcomes at the plan level.

References

Aizer, A., J. Currie, and E. Moretti. 2007. Does managed care hurt health? Evidence from Medicaid mothers. *Review of Economics and Statistics* 89, no. 3: 385-399.

Bella, M., C. Williams, L. Palmer, and S. Somers. 2006. *Seeking higher value in Medicaid: A national scan of state purchasers.* Hamilton NJ: Center for Health Care Strategies.

Bollinger, M.E., S.W. Smith, R. LoCasale, and C. Blaidsell. 2007. Transition to managed care impacts health care services utilization by children insured by Medicaid. *Journal of Asthma* 44, no. 9: 717-722.

Brown, R., J. Wooldridge, S. Hoag, and L. Moreno. 2001. *Reforming Medicaid: The experiences of five pioneering states with mandatory managed care and eligibility expansion. Report to the Health Care Financing Administration (now CMS) by Mathematica Policy Research,* contract no. 500-94-0047. http://www.mathematica-mpr.com/PDFs/reformmed.pdf.

California Health Care Foundation (CHCF). 2004. *Access to physicians in California's public insurance programs.* Issue brief. Oakland, CA: CHCF.

Centers for Medicare & Medicaid Services (CMS), Department of Health and Human Services. 2002. Medicaid program; Medicaid managed care: New provisions. Final rule. *Federal Register* 67, no. 115 (June 14): 40989-41038.

Chang, D., A. Burton, J. O'Brien, and R. Hurley. 2003. Honesty as good policy: Evaluating Maryland's Medicaid managed care program. *Milbank Quarterly* 81, no. 3.

Fontanella, C.A., S.J. Zuravin, and C.L. Burry. 2006. The effect of Medicaid managed care program on patterns of psychiatric readmission among adolescents: Evidence from Maryland. *Journal of Behavioral Health Services & Research* 33, no. 1: 39-52.

Gold, M., J. Mittler, D. Draper, and D. Rousseau. 2003. Participation of plans and providers in Medicaid and SCHIP managed care. *Health Affairs* 22, no.1: 230-240.

Gold, M., and A. Aizer. 2000. Growing an industry: How managed is TennCare's managed care? *Health Affairs* 19, no. 1: 86-101.

Gold, M. 1999. Medicaid managed care: Interpreting survey data within and across states. *Inquiry* 36(3): 332-342.

Government Accountability Office (GAO). 2009. *Medicaid preventive services: Concerted efforts needed to ensure beneficiaries receive services.* Washington, DC: GAO. http://www.gao.gov/new.items/d09578.pdf.

Kuhmerker, K., and T. Hartman. 2007. *Pay-for-performance in state Medicaid programs: A survey of state Medicaid directors and programs. Report to the Commonwealth Fund.* http://www.commonwealthfund.org/Content/Publications/Fund-Reports/2007/Apr/Pay-for-Performance-in-State-Medicaid-Programs--A-Survey-of-State-Medicaid-Directors-and-Programs.aspx.

Landon, B.E., and A. Epstein. 1999. Quality management practices in Medicaid managed care: A national survey of Medicaid and commercial health plans participating in the Medicaid program. *Journal of the American Medical Association* 282, no. 18: 1769-1775.

Lillie-Blanton, M., and B. Lyons. 1998. Managed care and low income populations: Recent state experiences. *Health Affairs* 17, no. 3: 238-247.

Long, S., and T. Coughlin. 2001. Impacts of Medicaid managed care on children. *Health Services Research* 36, no. 1: 7-23.

McCall, N. 1997. Lessons From Arizona's Medicaid Managed Care Program. *Health Affairs* 13, no.4: 194-199.

Medicaid and CHIP Payment and Access Commission (MACPAC). 2011. *March 2011 Report to the Congress on Medicaid and CHIP.* http://www.macpac.gov/reports.

Mitchell, J., K. Galina, and N. Swingonski. 2001. Impact of the Oregon Health Plan on children with special health care needs. *Pediatrics* 107, no.4: 736-743.

National Committee for Quality Assurance (NCQA). 2010a. *The state of health care quality: Reform, the quality agenda and resource use.* Washington, DC: NCQA. http://www.ncqa.org/portals/0/state%20of%20health%20care/2010/sohc%202010%20-%20full2.pdf.

National Committee for Quality Assurance (NCQA). 2010b. States using NCQA accreditation for Medicaid plans. http://www.ncqa.org/tabid/135/Default.aspx.

Rosenbaum, S., A. Markus, C. Sonosky, et al. 2003. *Accountability in Medicaid managed care: Implications for pediatric health care quality. Report to David and Lucile Packard Foundation.* http://www.gwumc.edu/sphhs/departments/healthpolicy/CHPR/downloads/Enforcement_12-2003.pdf.

Smith, V., K. Gifford, E. Ellis, et al. 2010. *Hoping for economic recovery, preparing for health reform: A look at Medicaid spending, coverage and policy trends.* Washington, DC: Kaiser Family Foundation (KFF). http://www.kff.org/medicaid/upload/8105.pdf.

Sparer, M. 2008. *Medicaid managed care reexamined.* New York, NY: Medicaid Institute at the United Hospital Funds. February.

URAC. 2009. *The URAC guide to Medicaid managed care external quality review.* http://www.urac.org/policyMakers/resources/URAC_Medicaid_EQR_Guide_INTRO_APP_A_and_B_2009.pdf.

Section E Annex

Preliminary Review of State Activities for Monitoring Access to Care

As a preliminary step in examining access to care in Medicaid, the Commission asked state Medicaid Directors to complete an informal questionnaire about state efforts for assessing access in Medicaid. From November 2010 through April 2011, Medicaid Directors in 47 states and the District of Columbia provided information about current activities for monitoring and identifying potential problems with access to care and provider capacity in their Medicaid programs.[1]

Examples of Access Monitoring by States

States indicated that they used many approaches to monitor access.

Monitoring enrollee feedback and conducting community outreach

▷ Monitor complaints through the use of enrollee or provider telephone hotlines

▷ Communicate regularly with a network of health care system stakeholders (i.e., beneficiary representatives, providers, local social service agencies, county case workers, public officials such as legislators or the Governor's office)

▷ Conduct community outreach with providers and beneficiary representatives

▷ Work with professional associations to encourage provider participation

Reviewing available data

▷ Review utilization data from the Medicaid Management Information System (MMIS) or a utilization dashboard to identify unusual patterns in claims and encounter data (i.e., use of emergency departments)

▷ Include requirements in managed care plan contracts for plans to measure and monitor access standards and report outcomes to the state on a prescribed schedule

▷ Require managed care plans to administer HEDIS and CAHPS data to monitor health plan performance on access as well as quality issues

▷ Analyze reports from transportation brokers to identify information on sudden changes in frequency or distance of transports

---

[1] All states and DC responded to the Commission's request for information; three states indicated that they were unable to complete the questionnaire at that time.

Leveraging other resources

▶ Work with academic institutions or other organizations in the state to monitor access-related issues

▶ Require managed care plans to sponsor initiatives to improve access when plans report access issues to the state as part of their contract requirements

▶ Hold managed care plans accountable for adjusting their networks, such as through the development of corrective action plans, if access issues arise

Examples of Provider Supply Monitoring by States

States use many techniques to monitor provider supply.

Reviewing available data

▶ Compare lists of participating providers to licensed providers

▶ Compare the location of participating providers to the location of beneficiaries

▶ Use Health Resources and Services Administration (HRSA) definitions to identify provider shortages

▶ Administer physician workforce surveys and surveys of primary and specialty providers to determine the Medicaid share of patients

▶ Analyze MMIS quarterly reports on primary and specialty care providers

▶ Assess whether providers listed in a managed care plan's network actually accept new patients

▶ Monitor compliance with standards specified in managed care plan contracts, including network adequacy, provider-to-patient ratios, and geo-access analysis

Leveraging other resources

▶ Work with sister agencies to monitor provider shortage areas

▶ Require managed care plans to compare the number of providers enrolled in Medicaid to the number of licensed providers or report on the prevalence of specific services such as emergency department care

SECTION

Program Accountability, Integrity, and Data

Federal and state spending on Medicaid and CHIP total more than $400 billion a year, accounting for more than 15 percent of U.S. health care spending (MACPAC 2011). Given the magnitude of these programs, federal and state governments have a statutory obligation to know whether or not they are paying appropriately for quality care and whether enrollees have adequate access to necessary care.

For states seeking to use managed care in their Medicaid programs, the federal government sets broad operational and administrative requirements related to payment rates to providers, provider availability in the plan network, provision of covered health care services, and quality of care for enrollees. Within these parameters states have flexibility in how they design and administer their programs and monitor participating plans. Subject to federal approval, states determine what covered services should be the responsibility of the managed care plans, which Medicaid enrollees should have managed care as an option, and whether enrollment is mandatory or voluntary. Both the federal and state agencies that oversee Medicaid are responsible for ensuring that mechanisms are in place to assure appropriate use of services and to detect and deter fraud, waste, and abuse.

This section describes:

▷ broad federal authority and program accountability requirements in states' Medicaid managed care programs;

▷ federal and state tools to improve program integrity; and

▷ some of the available data used for program accountability and integrity, and the data limitations that can hamper those efforts.

Broad Federal Authorities for Managed Care in Medicaid

States can implement managed care in their Medicaid programs under multiple federal authorities (Box F-1). The Social Security Act (the Act) allows states to mandate managed care enrollment and to waive certain other federal Medicaid requirements through a program waiver, a demonstration waiver, or a state plan amendment.[1] Twenty states and the District of Columbia now operate at least some aspect of their managed care program using this state plan option—up from 10 states in 2002 (KCMU 2010). For additional details on Medicaid managed care waiver and state plan authorities, see Table FA-1 in Section F Annex 1 of this Report.

Program Accountability

In order to receive federal Medicaid funds, states must meet numerous requirements regarding the proper and efficient administration of their Medicaid programs, including states' use of managed care in Medicaid. Over time, as the Congress has altered federal Medicaid law to provide new flexibilities for states' use of managed care, it has also added provisions to ensure that the federal government holds states accountable and that the states hold managed care plans accountable for the services they have agreed to provide to enrollees.

Under fee-for-service (FFS) Medicaid, the state pays providers directly for the services they provide. Under managed care, states often pay plans a fixed amount and allow the plans to pay providers a negotiated rate. Doing so, however, does not permit the state to shift to plans its federally mandated responsibility to ensure appropriate payment, access, and quality as required under federal law and regulations.

Indeed, the use of managed care brings some additional responsibilities to the state. The state must now ensure its contracts with plans meet relevant federal requirements and that appropriate safeguards are put in place for monitoring plan performance. In addition, as states move to managed care, the skill sets of staff may need to change. For additional details on managed care contracts, see Section F Annex 2 of this Report.

Key Federal Program Accountability Requirements in Managed Care

Federal law stipulates that states can receive federal Medicaid reimbursement for their payments to Medicaid managed care entities only if their contracts include certain provisions.[2] Federal statutory requirements on state contracts with these plans include, but are not limited to, the following (§1903(m)(2)(A)):

- The federal Department of Health and Human Services (HHS) and the state shall have the right to audit and inspect any books and records of the entity.

- The plan may not discriminate on the basis of enrollees' health status.

- Individuals can disenroll within the first 90 days without cause and then at least every 12 months thereafter.

---

[1] The Balanced Budget Act of 1997 (P.L. 105-33) gave state Medicaid programs the authority to mandate managed care enrollment without a waiver, except for certain children with special needs, Medicare beneficiaries, and American Indians. There are also federal requirements related to the enrollment of American Indians into Medicaid managed care. For example, a state may not require tribal members to enroll in managed care or a PCCM program, except when the entity is the Indian Health Service; an Indian health program operated by a tribe or a tribal organization pursuant to a contract, grant, cooperative agreement, or compact with the Indian Health Service; or an urban Indian health program operated by an urban Indian organization pursuant to a grant or contract with the Indian Health Service.

[2] See §1903(m)(2)(A) of the Act. This subparagraph also links to applicable requirements of §1932 per §1903(m)(2)(A)(xii).

BOX F-1. Key Federal Medicaid Managed Care Waiver Authorities

Section 1115 Research and Demonstration Waivers (17 states)	Allows states to test an "experimental, pilot, or demonstration project likely to assist in promoting the objectives of the programs" covered by the Social Security Act, including:

    ▷ Waiving statewideness requirements related to eligibility, benefits, and service delivery and payment methods used by the state to administer the managed care program.

    ▷ Identifying savings in the demonstrations to offset the cost of any program change, which can include managed care savings, to maintain budget neutrality.

Section 1915(b) Managed Care/Freedom of Choice Waivers (25 states)	Allows states to implement managed care and to limit individuals' choice of providers under Medicaid. States can also:

    ▷ Waive statewideness requirements (e.g., provide primary care case management or comprehensive risk-based managed care in a limited geographic area).

    ▷ Waive comparability requirements (e.g., provide enhanced benefits to managed care enrollees).

Combined Section 1915(b)/(c) Waivers (8 states)	Allows states to use two waiver authorities to provide home and community-based services to elderly or disabled Medicaid populations through their managed care programs, or to use a limited pool of providers to provide these services.

Some states use combined 1915(b)/(c) waivers to implement limited-benefit plans for specific services, such as prepaid inpatient health plans for behavioral health services. Other states use these waivers to provide integrated acute and long-term care services through a managed care delivery system for elderly and/or disabled Medicaid populations.

To implement concurrent 1915(b)/(c) waivers, states must meet all federal requirements, such as cost neutrality in the 1915(c) and cost effectiveness in the 1915(b) waiver.

Note: Section 1915(c) Home and Community-Based Services waivers allow states to provide home and community-based services as an alternative to institutional care in nursing homes, intermediate care facilities for the mentally retarded (ICFs/MR), and hospitals. States can provide targeted sets of services to specific populations including, for example, people with physical disabilities or HIV/AIDS, people with developmental disabilities, and people with traumatic brain injuries.

Source: The number of states operating managed care waivers from CMS 2010

▷ The plan must maintain patient encounter data and provide the data to the state at a frequency and level of detail specified by HHS.

In addition to states' own provisions to address plans' noncompliance, federal law stipulates that if a plan fails to provide the agreed-upon medically necessary services, charges premiums in excess of those permitted, or incurs other specified violations, the HHS Secretary may impose certain penalties, "in addition to any other remedies available under law." These include civil monetary penalties on the plan, as well as denial of federal Medicaid payments to the state for amounts paid under the contract (§1903(m)(5)(B)).

As discussed in greater detail in Section F Annex 2 of this Report, federal requirements related to states' contracts with plans pertain to the adequacy of provider networks, actuarial soundness, and other requirements. States are often given considerable flexibility in how they operationalize these requirements and determine how the plans meet them. For example, states vary considerably in how they measure, monitor, and evaluate the adequacy of provider networks. Common requirements include specific enrollee-to-provider ratios, travel time and distance standards, and other metrics such as wait times for appointments. States may require managed care plans to submit routine network adequacy reports (e.g., updated ratios, provider panel status, geographic analyses) or ad hoc data in the event of a suspected network access issue.

To establish an adequate network, plans must consider:

- anticipated Medicaid enrollment;
- expected service use, taking into consideration the specific characteristics and health needs of the Medicaid enrollees who will be enrolled in the plan;
- the number and types of providers required to provide the contracted services;
- the number of network providers who are not accepting new Medicaid patients; and
- the geographic location of providers and Medicaid enrollees, considering distance, travel time, the means of transportation generally used by Medicaid enrollees, and whether the location provides physical access for Medicaid enrollees with disabilities.

Other examples of federal managed care requirements include:

- standards for timely access to care and services, taking into account the urgency of the need for such services;
- network providers who offer hours of operation that are no fewer than the hours of operation offered to commercial enrollees or comparable to Medicaid FFS providers;
- making contracted services available 24 hours a day, seven days a week, when medically necessary; and
- mechanisms to ensure compliance by providers through monitoring and applying corrective actions for noncompliance.

States are required to provide enrollees and prospective enrollees with information explaining the managed care program, including basic features such as benefits covered, cost sharing and carve outs, and populations excluded or exempted from managed care enrollment (42 CFR 438.10).

Federal requirements also address enrollees' rights (42 CFR 438 Subpart C). Plans must have written policies regarding enrollees' rights, including but not limited to receipt of easily understood materials and information on treatment options and alternatives, participation in health care decisions, request and receipt of personal medical records, and ability to receive health care services in accordance with federal laws. All information such as enrollment notices and instructional materials must be communicated in a manner and format that is easily understood and takes into consideration the special needs of the certain populations (e.g., persons with limited vision or those with limited reading proficiency).

In addition, federal regulations (42 CFR 438 Subparts D-E) provide states with a baseline set of requirements for monitoring and assessing the quality of care provided to Medicaid managed care enrollees. States are required to have in place strategies for monitoring plans' quality and performance in order to assess the quality and appropriateness of care and services provided to all Medicaid enrollees under managed care contracts. For example, as described in Section E of this Report, many states require plans to provide quality and performance measures from the Healthcare Effectiveness Data and Information Set (HEDIS)[3] and the Consumer Assessment of Healthcare Providers and Systems (CAHPS).[4] Although there is an effort underway for states to report such measures voluntarily to the federal government for children enrolled in Medicaid and CHIP, results are not currently available for cross-state comparisons of Medicaid managed care programs.

States must also require each plan to have an ongoing quality and performance improvement program for the services it provides to its enrollees. At least annually states must review the impact and effectiveness of each plan's quality assessment and performance improvement program. Finally, each state must ensure that a qualified external quality review organization (EQRO) performs an annual external quality review (EQR) for each contracting plan. States are required to report to CMS the EQRO's validation of certain measures, not the results of the measures themselves. Moreover, an analysis by CMS found that states' EQROs used a variety of measures such that no nationally standardized information is currently available from EQROs (HHS 2010).

Program Integrity

As an integral component of program accountability, program integrity (PI) efforts seek to ensure proper payment for appropriate, high quality services in both FFS and managed care. This includes addressing not only fraud, waste, and abuse by providers and enrollees, but also program management issues.

Federal Program Integrity Efforts

To address concerns about the program's vulnerability to financial losses and previously low levels of resources devoted to PI, the Congress has provided new requirements and funding for these activities in recent years. The Deficit Reduction Act of 2005 (P.L. 109-171) provided additional dedicated funding for Medicaid PI activities, including the establishment of a Medicaid Integrity Program (MIP), which supports states in their efforts to combat fraud, waste, and abuse. MIP also conducts provider audits, identifies overpayments, and educates providers and others about PI issues.

The Patient Protection and Affordable Care Act (PPACA, P.L. 111-148) created additional requirements to increase uniformity and improve Medicaid PI activities. These efforts include additional provider screening requirements, creating an integrated Medicare and Medicaid data repository to enhance data sharing among federal and state agencies and law enforcement officials, requiring states to contract with recovery audit contractors to identify underpayments and overpayments and to recoup overpayments, and strengthening requirements related to the termination of providers participating in Medicaid if they have been terminated under Medicare or other state health care programs.

---

[3] HEDIS is a registered trademark of the National Committee for Quality Assurance (NCQA).

[4] CAHPS is a registered trademark of the Agency for Healthcare Research and Quality, which oversees the survey.

State Program Integrity Efforts

State efforts to address PI issues include both designing and managing Medicaid programs to prevent fraud, waste, and abuse and also having appropriate systems in place to identify problems when they occur. Program management efforts can include, for example, data systems coordination to prevent inappropriate payments for their enrollees in managed care (e.g., not paying FFS claims for an enrollee who is in managed care or not making capitation payments to multiple plans for one enrollee).

Program integrity efforts also include utilization management, such as requiring prior authorization of certain services, prospective and retrospective service reviews, and outreach to providers and enrollees to correct inappropriate utilization practices. Because Medicaid is the payer of last resort, PI also includes taking reasonable measures to determine legal liability of third parties and, if third party liability (TPL) exists, attempting to ensure that the provider bills the third party before sending the claim to Medicaid or recovering money from the third party when the state discovers it has paid a claim in error (42 CFR 433.138).

As part of federal efforts to identify improper payments,[5] states must submit information to CMS for estimating improper payments in the FFS and managed care components of their Medicaid program and determining whether eligibility decisions were made correctly. This process, known as Payment Error Rate Measurement (PERM), uses a statistically valid random sample of claims and eligibility determinations to determine error rates.[6] Each state must develop a corrective action plan to reduce improper payments based on the error causes identified and is required to return the federal share of overpayments to CMS (42 CFR 431 Subpart Q).

A state's ability to detect fraud and abuse once it has occurred requires adequate data and information, including encounter data. Under federal regulations, states must have methods and criteria for identifying suspected fraud and abuse. They must have established procedures for affording due process and for protecting the legal rights of those involved, but also for referring cases to law enforcement officials when appropriate (42 CFR 455.13).

Upon receipt of a complaint of fraud or abuse or identification of questionable practices, the state Medicaid agency must conduct a preliminary investigation. If there is a sufficient basis to warrant a full investigation, depending on the circumstances, the agency may conduct the investigation itself, refer the case to the Medicaid Fraud Control Unit (MFCU),[7] or to the appropriate law enforcement agency. An investigation will continue until appropriate legal action is initiated, the case is closed or dropped because of insufficient evidence, or the matter has been resolved between the agency and the individual or entity under investigation (42 CFR 455.14-16).

As a way to initially screen and provide ongoing monitoring of providers, the Medicaid state plan must ensure that providers and fiscal agents disclose certain information for each person with at least a 5 percent ownership or controlling interest in the entity and agree to provide information related to business transactions upon request (42 CFR 455 Subpart B).

---

[5] Improper payments are defined as any payment that should not have been made or that was made in an incorrect amount. The Improper Payments Information Act of 2002 (P.L. 107-300) requires federal agencies to review and identify annually those programs and activities that may be susceptible to significant erroneous payments, estimate the amount of improper payments, report such estimates to the Congress, and submit a report on actions the agency is taking to reduce erroneous payments.

[6] PERM is usually conducted on a rotating basis in 17 states annually.

[7] MFCUs investigate and prosecute Medicaid fraud, as well as review complaints of abuse and neglect in health care facilities.

Managed Care Plan Program Integrity Efforts

In states with managed care programs, PI efforts extend to the plans, as they are required to follow all applicable federal and state PI requirements. States generally include specific PI requirements in their contracts with plans. Although states monitor plan PI efforts, plans have their own incentives to identify and address possible fraud and abuse because they are paid a capitated rate for each enrollee in their plan. In the event that there is undetected fraud, waste, and abuse in managed care, however, this cost could be passed on to the state in the form of increased future capitation payments.

Data for Program Accountability and Policy Development

Data reported by managed care plans and states provide important information for answering key policy and program accountability questions. For example, data are necessary to monitor trends and make projections on spending, service use, and the quality and appropriateness of care. However, data submitted by managed care plans to states and by states to CMS vary in their consistency, availability, and timeliness. This variability creates challenges for analyzing and monitoring managed care programs and limits the ability to compare states. Section 4 of MACStats provides more information on issues that should be noted when examining managed care statistics from different data sources.

Managed Care Encounter Data

All states that contract with managed care plans collect encounter data that provide a record of the services furnished to Medicaid enrollees. However, many states do not report these data to the federal government in the Medicaid Statistical Information System (MSIS) as required (OIG 2009). Among states that do report encounter data in MSIS, the quality of the data are largely unknown. CMS recently began a project to explore this issue and provide technical assistance to states. It is also developing a regulation on the submission of encounter data in MSIS. As discussed in MACPAC's March 2011 Report to the Congress, these data could be used for a number of purposes, including national and cross-state comparisons of the care received by enrollees in FFS versus managed care systems—which some states already do on an individual basis.

Managed Care Enrollment Report

States report information on their managed care programs through the Medicaid Managed Care Data Collection System (MMCDCS). From this, CMS produces an annual Medicaid Managed Care Enrollment Report that provides national, regional, and state-level point-in-time enrollment statistics for enrollees in managed care programs of various types (CMS 2010).[8] In addition to higher-level enrollment data, this report also includes the following plan-specific data: plan name, managed care entity, reimbursement arrangement, operating authority, geographic area served, number of enrollees by plan, and number of dual eligibles by plan.

---

[8] Reports are based on data for June 30 of each year.

Medicaid Statistical Information System (MSIS)

MSIS is a data source compiled by CMS from detailed eligibility and claims information reported by all states since FY 1999. Previously, states were only required to provide aggregate statistics on Medicaid enrollment, service use, and spending in an annual report. States now must submit five MSIS files every quarter: one file containing eligibility-related information on each person enrolled in the state Medicaid program (e.g., months of Medicaid enrollment, basis of eligibility, dual enrollment in Medicare, demographics such as age, sex, and race/ethnicity), and four files containing information on paid claims for inpatient hospital, institutional long-term care, drugs, and other services (e.g., type of service, place of service, amount paid by Medicaid, and diagnoses).

With regard to managed care, MSIS contains the following information for each enrollee:

▶ plan ID numbers and types for up to four managed care plans under which the enrollee is covered during each month;

▶ the waiver ID number, if enrolled in a Section 1915(b) or other waiver;

▶ claims that provide a record of each capitated payment made on behalf of the enrollee to a managed care plan, which are generally referred to as capitated claims; and

▶ claims that provide a record of each service received by the enrollee from a provider under contract with a managed care plan, which generally do not include a payment amount and are referred to as encounter or "dummy" claims. As noted earlier, all states collect encounter data from their Medicaid managed care plans, but some do not report it in MSIS.

References

Centers for Medicare & Medicaid Services (CMS), Department of Health and Human Services. 2010. *2009 National Summary of State Medicaid Managed Care Programs*. Washington, DC: HHS. https://www.cms.gov/MedicaidDataSourcesGenInfo/downloads/2009NationalSummaryReport.pdf.

Department of Health and Human Services (HHS). 2010. *The Department of Health and Human Services Children's Health Insurance Program Reauthorization Act annual report on the quality of care for children in Medicaid and CHIP*. Washington, DC: HHS. http://www.cms.gov/MedicaidCHIPQualPrac/Downloads/secrep.pdf.

Kaiser Commission on Medicaid and the Uninsured (KCMU). 2010. *Medicaid and managed care: Key data, trends, and issues*. Washington, DC: KCMU. http://www.kff.org/medicaid/upload/8046.pdf.

Medicaid and CHIP Payment and Access Commission (MACPAC). 2011. *March 2011 Report to the Congress on Medicaid and CHIP*. http://www.macpac.gov/reports.

Office of the Inspector General (OIG), Department of Health and Human Services. 2009. *Medicaid managed care encounter data: collection and use*. Washington, DC: OIG. http://oig.hhs.gov/oei/reports/oei-07-06-00540.pdf.

Section F Annex 1

Key Federal Authorities Allowing Medicaid Managed Care

The Social Security Act (the Act) provides multiple authorities under which states may operate Medicaid managed care programs (with federal approval)—through a state plan amendment (SPA), Section 1915(b) program waiver, or a Section 1115 research and demonstration waiver. These authorities differ in what options they allow states to use in the design of their managed care programs, including populations enrolled, service delivery, and benefits covered, as well as in the processes for CMS review and approval of the proposed managed care program. Table FA-1 below highlights key features of each authority.

TABLE FA-1. Characteristics of Key Medicaid Managed Care SPAs and Waivers

	1932(a) SPAs	Section 1915(b) Program Waivers	Section 1115 Research and Demonstration Waivers
General Authority	Exempts states from state plan requirements for: • **Statewideness** (i.e., managed care program does not have to be operational statewide) • **Comparability** (i.e., benefits for managed care enrollees can differ from those provided to non-managed care enrollees) • **Freedom of choice** (i.e., ability of enrollees to receive services from any qualified provider); used to require enrollment in a managed care program and limit choice of provider to those in the health plan's network.	Provides states a waiver from state plan requirements for: • **Statewideness** • **Comparability** • **Freedom of choice** Authority can also be used to provide additional services that are not otherwise provided to non-enrollees, as well as to limit the number of providers with which the state contracts to provide services.	Section 1115 authority is broad, potentially permitting all of the flexibility allowed under 1915(b) waivers as well as the waiver of other federal Medicaid requirements contained in Section 1902 of the Act. Further, under this authority, the Secretary can provide federal matching funds for services /activities/ costs not otherwise matchable (CNOM).

TABLE FA-1, Continued

	1932(a) SPAs	Section 1915(b) Program Waivers	Section 1115 Research and Demonstration Waivers
Approval Period[1]	Indefinite.	Initially approved for two years.	Initially approved for five years.
Populations That Can Be Mandatorily Enrolled	All state plan populations except certain children with special needs, Medicare beneficiaries, and American Indians.	All state plan populations.	All state plan populations, as well as any individuals not otherwise eligible for Medicaid (authorized through CNOM).
Application Requirements	Completion of mandatory CMS state plan preprint.	Completion of CMS application template.	No CMS standard preprint form or template available, but must submit proposal describing design features of program (e.g., populations covered, design of Medicaid managed care program).
Federal Budget Requirements	No required budget or cost analysis.	Demonstrate cost effectiveness and efficiency of program (actual expenditures cannot exceed projected expenditures for approval period).	Demonstrate budget neutrality (federal expenditures cannot be greater during the approval period with the waiver than without the waiver).
CMS Review Timeframe	Approved within 90 days of CMS receipt unless written disapproval or request for additional information. If additional information requested, 90-day period begins again on day CMS receives additional information.	Approved within 90 days of CMS receipt unless written disapproval or request for additional information. If additional information requested, 90-day period begins again on day CMS receives additional information.	No required timeframe for CMS review or approval.
Renewal Period[1]	No renewal needed.	Customarily up to two years; CMS has discretion to approve for five years if enrollees dually eligible for Medicare and Medicaid are served by the waiver.	Customarily up to three years; CMS has the discretion to approve for five years if enrollees dually eligible for Medicare and Medicaid are served by the waiver.

---

[1] Section 2601 of the Patient Protection and Affordable Care Act provides for a 5-year approval or renewal period for certain Medicaid waivers impacting demonstration programs under Section 1115 of the Act and waivers under Sections 1915(b) and 1915(c) of the Act, through which a state serves individuals who are dually eligible for Medicare and Medicaid. At the Secretary's discretion, a waiver that provides medical assistance for dually eligible beneficiaries can be approved for an initial period of up to 5 years and renewed for up to 5 years, at the state's request.

TABLE FA-1, Continued

	1932(a) SPAs	Section 1915(b) Program Waivers	Section 1115 Research and Demonstration Waivers
Program Documentation	Contained within overall CMS state plan preprint.	Contained within CMS application template.	Special terms and conditions negotiated between CMS and states and documented.
Monitoring/ Evaluation	CMS monitors implementation of SPA to ensure requirements are met; state required to conduct separate evaluation of managed care entities.	CMS monitors implementation of waiver to ensure requirements are met; state required to conduct separate evaluation of managed care entities.	CMS monitors implementation of waiver to ensure requirements are met; required periodic evaluation of the project (often conducted by the state).

Section F Annex 2

Comprehensive Risk-based Contract Requirements

The contractual obligations placed on managed care plans in Medicaid can be important to the success or failure of a Medicaid managed care program. Managed care provides states with an opportunity to delegate financial risk for the care of enrollees to participating plans. However, states are ultimately responsible for the performance of their Medicaid programs. Clearly outlined responsibilities and requirements, appropriate financing arrangements, and diligent oversight are essential to establishing an accountable and efficient program.

The contract constitutes a legal agreement between the state and a managed care plan for the delivery of services to enrollees and functions as a mechanism to enforce the standards specified by states and the federal government. Managed care plan contract terms and conditions vary among states in the level of specificity of plan requirements, but all include a basic set of activities, many mandated by federal law.[1] (In Sections E and F of this Report, we outline the federal requirements that serve as the basis for these contracting provisions.) Contracts and plan responsibilities are subject to CMS oversight, including review and approval by CMS staff. As states move to managed care, the staff skill sets may need to change.

Key elements of state managed care contracts may include, but are not limited to:

  ▸ **Network development and maintenance.** In comprehensive risk-based managed care programs, rather than dealing directly with individual providers, states delegate the responsibility of establishing and maintaining provider networks to the plans. To ensure that plans contract with a sufficient number and type of providers, including specialists, states often include network requirements in their plan contracts. Plans must also guarantee that providers meet certain credentialing requirements.

  ▸ **Care management and coordination.** States often require plans to assign each enrollee to a designated primary care provider who will coordinate an enrollee's care across providers and services. Plans may also be required to assign certain enrollees to care managers for additional assistance with the coordination of services

---

[1] Part 438 of the Code of Federal Regulations outlines the following managed care requirements: General Provisions, State Responsibilities, Enrollee Rights and Protection, Quality Assessment and Performance Improvement, External Quality Review, Grievance System, Certifications and Program Integrity, Sanctions, and Conditions for Federal Financial Participation.

as well as provide services such as general health education and disease management to enrollees.

▷ **Customer service and member education.** Plan contracts must ensure that enrollees receive necessary information about obtaining services and have a way to contact their respective plans with questions or concerns. Toll-free hotlines and ombudsman programs are commonly used tools.

▷ **Quality standards and reporting.** In addition to enforcing federal requirements for external quality reviews and reporting, states may also include their own requirements for ensuring that quality services are provided to enrollees. Section E of this Report provides additional information on the types of quality monitoring activities that Medicaid managed care plans are required to conduct as part of federal requirements.

▷ **Data collection.** States and the federal government have various data collection requirements that plans must comply with when serving Medicaid enrollees including but not limited to requirements on enrollment data, encounter data, and reporting of certain quality measures.

▷ **Monitoring and evaluation.** To determine if plans are meeting contract requirements, states monitor and evaluate plan performance. Some Medicaid programs are very prescriptive in the types and frequency of reports required from plans. Other states may have less structured contract requirements, allowing the state to request information from plans on an ad hoc basis.

▷ **Payment.** Capitation payment amounts are typically part of the contract language. Contracts also typically stipulate that plans have a specified amount of time to process claims and make payments to providers.[2] Contracts may also contain requirements and standards for reporting encounter and financial data to the state.

▷ **Corrective action.** The contract specifies how corrective action plans will be developed and implemented when issues or problems are identified with plan performance.

In addition to these areas, CMS regulations outline a number of other requirements that must be contained in plan contracts, such as compliance with federal and state contracting rules, inspection and audit of financial records, and prohibition of enrollment discrimination (42 CFR 438.6).

There is a wide range of variation in the level of detail of contract requirements across states and in the overall plan contracting process, and states may update their contracts as they learn more about effective contracting mechanisms to improve quality and oversight. There is currently no central source at the federal level that allows for the analysis of how states use the contracting process for program accountability in their Medicaid programs. This may also make comparisons to FFS difficult.

---

[2] Section 1902(a)(37)(A) of the Act requires that 90 percent of claims for services provided by health care providers under a managed care plan must be paid within 30 days of receipt and that 99 percent of claims are paid within 90 days of receipt.

SECTION

Issues Facing Medicaid and CHIP Managed Care

Medicaid managed care arrangements differ from those in the private sector and in Medicare in part due to differences in the populations served. Enrollment of low-income populations (e.g., at or below 133 percent of the federal poverty level or $24,645 a year for a family of three) with limited resources and often complex health needs affects Medicaid managed care program design. The role of provider networks, the use of cost sharing as a tool for managing utilization, the enrollment process and the types of organizations sponsoring managed care plans in different markets differ from private sector and Medicare managed care plans. These distinct differences can affect whether and how states use managed care in Medicaid to deliver quality care.

Managed care in Medicaid has taken on many forms: comprehensive risk-based plans, primary care case management (PCCM) programs, and limited-benefit plans. These arrangements are a major part of Medicaid programs in many states and their role is likely to expand over the coming years. In a recent survey, 20 states said they anticipated some expansion in Medicaid managed care in FY 2011 (Smith et al. 2010). While the focus of this report has been on Medicaid managed care, managed care plays a significant role in CHIP programs as well, though evaluation, analyses, and data are limited.

States have pursued managed care strategies as a way to improve care management and care coordination, secure provider networks for enrollees, lower spending or make it more predictable, and improve program accountability. All of these goals will continue to be important as states work to improve the health of Medicaid enrollees, both in managed care and fee for service (FFS), while addressing budget constraints. However, state strategies are likely to differ based on factors such as population characteristics, population density, provider availability, plan participation, state goals, and existing managed care arrangements in each state.

Managed Care in Medicaid Today

Since states first began testing managed care as a part of Medicaid in the early years of the program, much has changed. Approximately 49 million Medicaid enrollees receive care through some form of Medicaid managed care. This Report presents the current status of managed care in Medicaid as it continues to evolve. As this Report shows, at this point in the evolution of Medicaid managed care:

Trends in Enrollment (See MACStats Tables 9 and 11). Comprehensive risk-based managed care enrollment in Medicaid is growing nationwide, and the population covered is expanding to enrollees with disabilities.

▶ Medicaid enrollment in comprehensive risk-based programs has increased to 47 percent of enrollees in 2009, up from 15 percent in 1995.

▶ Low-income children and non-disabled adults under age 65 were most likely to be enrolled in comprehensive risk-based managed care (60 percent and 44 percent respectively) in FY 2008 than other groups.

▶ Individuals with disabilities were enrolled in comprehensive risk-based programs in 39 states and the District of Columbia in FY 2008; 28 percent of all Medicaid enrollees with disabilities are enrolled in comprehensive risk-based managed care. However, the percentage of this group's enrollment in comprehensive risk-based managed care varies significantly by state—from less than 1 percent to over 90 percent.

▶ Low-income individuals age 65 and older, mostly with primary coverage through Medicare, were the least likely to be enrolled in comprehensive risk-based managed care:

11 percent of all Medicaid enrollees age 65 and older were enrolled in comprehensive risk-based managed care programs in FY 2008.

Managed Care Arrangements (See MACStats Table 9 and 10). States choose managed care arrangements and/or FFS depending on their unique populations, provider base, benefits, geography, and state goals.

▶ Thirty-four states and the District of Columbia had comprehensive risk-based Medicaid managed care programs with 21 states and the District of Columbia enrolling more than half of their total Medicaid population in such programs.[1] Many of the 16 states without comprehensive risk-based plans are largely rural.

▶ Thirty states used PCCM programs to coordinate care in FFS and 34 states and the District of Columbia used limited-benefit plans to provide selected services (such as behavioral health and oral health) in managed care and FFS settings.

▶ Thirty-seven states and the District of Columbia used a combination of two or more managed care arrangements and 13 states used all three managed care approaches in their Medicaid programs.[2]

▶ Using the CMS definition, 71 percent of Medicaid enrollees in FY 2009 were enrolled in some form of managed care in 48 states and the District of Columbia. Most Medicaid enrollees still receive at least some services through FFS arrangements.

---

[1] Seven additional states have Program for All-inclusive Care for the Elderly (PACE) programs but no other comprehensive risk-based managed care.

[2] Excludes PACE programs.

Payment Policy. There is considerable variation in the way states pay managed care plans.

▷ States with comprehensive risk-based managed care generally use forms of administered pricing or competitive bidding to establish payment rates for plans. Rates are required to be actuarially sound.

▷ States use different methods of adjusting payments to reflect the health and demographic characteristics of enrollees. More work is needed on risk adjustment models for complex, low-income populations.

▷ For some states, moving populations into managed care has implications for certain supplemental payments.

Access, Quality, and Program Accountability. Monitoring program integrity, quality, and access to care is challenging due to a lack of data and up to date analyses.

▷ The consistency, availability, and timeliness of the data submitted by managed care plans to states and subsequently from states to CMS vary considerably, creating challenges for analyzing and monitoring managed care programs and policies at the national level. This limits the ability to create baseline data and compare states.

▷ Multistate data and analyses on managed care arrangements would better enable monitoring of program integrity, appropriate utilization of health care services, and access to care.

Current and Future Issues

In this context of existing growth and variety in managed care arrangements, three overarching questions exist for policymakers as managed care continues to evolve in Medicaid and CHIP:

1. How can current managed care programs in Medicaid be improved for the low-income

populations currently served? How can these lessons be applied to CHIP?

2. How can care management best address the high health care needs and costs of low-income populations including children with special health care needs, individuals with disabilities, and dual eligibles who are increasingly likely to be enrolled in managed care in the future?

3. How can managed care meet the needs of new adult populations potentially enrolling in Medicaid starting in 2014?

Key issues stemming from these three questions include: enrollment, plan participation, benefit design, payment, access to care and care quality, and data for program accountability and program integrity. Building on the baseline information in this Report, the Commission will seek to provide a better understanding of these issues as the basis for future work on how health care delivery and financing can work even more effectively for Medicaid and CHIP enrollees.

Enrollees

Historically, the Medicaid managed care environment has primarily focused on children and parents, but increasingly states are moving to cover enrollees with more complex health care needs to manage costs and improve care management. With implementation of the Patient Protection and Affordable Care Act (PPACA, P.L. 111-148), the populations that states seek to enroll in managed care will increase further.

Much more could be known about what program features work best for different populations, and how to adapt managed care programs as states continue to extend them to additional populations. For example, individuals with complex, chronic medical needs may benefit from particular methods of care management and may need a different mix of providers in a provider network. Individuals dually eligible for coverage through Medicare and Medicaid bring an additional set of complexities because of the need to coordinate with benefits covered and financed by the Medicare program.

States may also need to fine-tune their existing managed care enrollment processes to serve an increasing—and increasingly diverse—number of enrollees in managed care. For example, to ensure continuity of services and coordination of benefits, mandatory enrollment and auto-assignment processes might differ for enrollees with disabilities as compared with the processes states have typically used for low-income children and families. In addition, the health insurance exchanges expected to be implemented in 2014 will likely change program enrollment for Medicaid and CHIP because states are required to create an eligibility and enrollment process that integrates Medicaid and CHIP with the exchanges. Under current law, income eligibility levels for Medicaid will rise to 138 percent of poverty[3] ($15,028 for one person) for most adults in 2014—an expansion of Medicaid to new groups of eligibles in most states. This will be a diverse group, ranging from healthy young adults to older low-income individuals with multiple chronic conditions. Many of these newly eligible individuals will have little to no experience with Medicaid or other forms of health insurance.

The use of managed care for these new Medicaid enrollees will undoubtedly continue to vary substantially across the country as states adopt arrangements that meet their particular environments and state goals. For states that are already experienced with rate setting and contracting issues in comprehensive risk-based managed care arrangements, enrolling additional populations into comprehensive risk-based plans represents more of an incremental change. Other states with less managed care experience or capacity may find it easier to continue to rely on FFS or arrangements like PCCM to serve these additional enrollees.

One additional consideration for states is how to manage care for a population whose incomes fluctuate from month to month. A recent study estimated that under the new eligibility rules, as many as half of adults with incomes under 200 percent of poverty ($21,780 for one person)— approximately 28 million people—can be expected to experience changes in income that could change their Medicaid eligibility status within a single year (Sommers and Rosenbaum 2011). In this respect, these new eligibles will be similar to the non-disabled adults under age 65 who are currently enrolled in Medicaid, who are covered on average for just two-thirds of the year (Ku et al. 2009). This level of turnover will continue to be a challenge for states and plans seeking to manage care for part-year enrollees.

Plan Types and Benefit Designs

The Medicaid managed care market is a mix of comprehensive risk-based plans (in 34 states plus the District of Columbia), PCCM programs (in 30 states), and limited-benefit plans (in 34 states plus the District of Columbia). All but two states use at least one of these arrangements, and 13 states use all three types of managed care (MACStats Table 10). Because insurance markets vary from state to state, arrangements that work best for Medicaid managed care or even for a certain type of enrollee are likely to vary across states. Policymakers would benefit, however, from more systematic analyses of how use of different managed care models

---

[3] For individuals whose eligibility is determined using modified adjusted gross income starting in 2014, the eligibility limit is 133 percent of the federal poverty level (FPL), plus states will apply an income disregard equal to 5 percent of the FPL. This means that an individual whose total income equals 138 percent of the FPL will only have 133 percent of the FPL counted when his or her Medicaid eligibility is determined.

and types of plans affect costs and outcomes for different populations. For example, states have very different experiences with carving out benefits from comprehensive risk-based managed care plans, but little research has been done on the effects of those different carve-out policies.

The landscape of comprehensive risk-based plan sponsors across the overall health system is likely to change with the introduction of insurance exchanges under PPACA, with potential ripple effects on plan participation in Medicaid and CHIP managed care. Concurrent with these changes, states and other players in the health care arena will likely continue to explore new options for care management outside the context of the managed care plans that exist today, including employing new models such as health homes and accountable care organizations (ACOs).

Payment

Payments for both FFS and managed care are likely to be under fiscal pressure as states continue to struggle with budget challenges. Some states may seek additional savings through experimenting with delivery models such as ACOs and health homes; others may focus on lowering costs for existing managed care programs or moving enrollees into managed care.

States' ability to find savings through managed care may vary depending on the availability of providers, the existing practice patterns of those providers, the patterns of service use by Medicaid and CHIP enrollees, and current FFS payment levels. For example, plans in states with a large number of providers likely have more capacity to establish networks and negotiate payment rates than do plans in states with provider shortages. Factors such as these will affect states' decisions on which kinds of managed care to pursue or whether to pursue managed care at all.

Much more could be known about how states set payment rates and use risk adjustment and risk sharing. Many states with more mature risk-based managed care systems, and particularly those that have moved to enroll high need populations such as individuals with disabilities, have developed systems to adjust plan payments based on the health status of low-income enrollees. However, there is no comprehensive source of information on the methodologies states use to risk adjust their managed care payments. Other states have not yet worked out the payment issues for these more complex, higher cost populations.

Access and Quality

Under both FFS and managed care arrangements in Medicaid and CHIP, enrollee access to appropriate services and care quality will be ongoing issues. Although many states have systems for monitoring the impact of Medicaid managed care on access to providers, use of services, and quality, systematic studies are limited and dated. Collecting more recent evidence across states will help inform both state and federal policymakers about the impact of managed care on access to appropriate care and cost for serving vulnerable populations.

Improved information and analyses would inform the assessment of access to care over time in both FFS and managed care.

Program Accountability

CMS sets broad operational and administrative requirements but gives states flexibility in how they determine operational methods, contract with plans, administer the program, and monitor participating plans. Federal and state agencies overseeing the Medicaid and CHIP programs are responsible for ensuring that mechanisms to promote access, quality, and program efficiency are in place to prevent fraud, waste, and abuse and to identify problems when they occur.

Contracting with managed care plans may shift some responsibilities in these areas onto the plans, but it also creates new responsibilities for states. When states move from primarily staffing for FFS claims processing and operations to staffing to implement managed care programs by contracting with plans, new staff skill sets are often required to focus on plan oversight and monitoring.

Federal and state oversight of managed care in Medicaid and CHIP likely will continue to change as these programs evolve. For example, CMS is currently working with states to improve the submission of encounter data from comprehensive risk-based plans. As enrollment in managed care continues to grow, this will be an essential source of information not only for program accountability but also for research on other issues related to access and quality.

Data

Evaluating managed care's impact on access, quality, and program spending at the national level is limited by lack of timely and accurate data. Data already exist in many states, but they generally are not standardized or gathered together in a way that facilitates analyses across states. Most research examining managed care in Medicaid and CHIP is old and thus less relevant to current programs. For populations currently enrolled in managed care and for those likely to be enrolled in the future, it will be essential to improve the data available at both the state and the national level to address policy questions and provide timely program assessments.

Next Steps

The Congress established MACPAC as a nonpartisan advisor to provide technical and analytic assistance, and to be a source of current, reliable information to guide policies related to Medicaid and CHIP. MACPAC's future analytic agenda will continue to focus on managed care as well as FFS in these programs.

Just as this Report has looked at the evolution of managed care in Medicaid, in the future MACPAC will look at the evolution of managed care in CHIP. Children in stand-alone CHIP programs are even more likely than children in Medicaid to be enrolled in managed care: 81 percent are enrolled in a comprehensive risk-based managed care plan. Analyzing how managed care is working across states and for diverse populations in both Medicaid and CHIP will help state and federal policymakers understand how programs can be improved to promote appropriate access and quality while controlling costs.

Managed care currently plays a central role in many state Medicaid programs, with nearly half of all enrollees nationwide in comprehensive risk-based plans. That role may broaden in the future, as states consider managed care arrangements to cover a more diverse mix of low-income enrollees including high need, high cost populations. Moving forward, states will continue to evaluate which managed care or FFS arrangements work best for their populations now and in the future.

References

Ku, L., P. MacTaggart, F. Pervez, and S. Rosenbaum. 2009. *Improving Medicaid's continuity of coverage and quality of care. Report to the Association for Community Affiliated Plans.* Washington, DC: George Washington University Department of Health Policy. http://www.ahcahp.org/Portals/0/ACAP%20Docs/Improving%20Medicaid%20Final%20070209.pdf.

Smith, V., K. Gifford, E. Ellis, et al. 2010. *Hoping for economic recovery, preparing for health reform: A look at Medicaid spending, coverage and policy trends.* Washington, DC: Kaiser Family Foundation (KFF). http://www.kff.org/medicaid/upload/8105.pdf.

Sommers, B.D., and S. Rosenbaum. 2011. Issues in health reform: How changes in eligibility may move millions back and forth between Medicaid and insurance exchanges. *Health Affairs* 30, no. 4: 228-236.

Medicaid and CHIP Program Statistics: June 2011 MACStats

Updated on July 25, 2011, Tables 4B, 5A, and 5B reflect corrections to typographical errors found after the Report's publication. As a result, some numbers in these tables differ from those in the published report. Tables 6, 7, and 11 each reflect the addition of a clarifying footnote after the Report's publication.

MACStats Table of Contents

MACStats

Overview of MACStats

MACStats is a standing section in all MACPAC reports to the Congress. It was created because data and information on the Medicaid and CHIP programs can often be difficult to find and are spread out across a variety of sources. The June 2011 edition of MACStats illustrates trends in Medicaid enrollment and spending, as well as health and other characteristics, service use, and spending among Medicaid and CHIP populations. It also supplements the Report's Medicaid managed care sections with state-level data on Medicaid managed care plans, enrollment, and spending.

In addition to state-level data by eligibility group, data highlighting users of long-term services and supports (LTSS) and other enrollee subgroups such as children with special health care needs are presented. These data illustrate how specific Medicaid populations differ in terms of their characteristics, service use, and spending.

Medicaid and CHIP serve a variety of low-income populations (Tables 9, 10, and 11 in the March 2011 MACStats), including non-disabled children and adults who account for a large share of program enrollment—nearly 75 percent of all Medicaid enrollees in FY 2008. Many of the June 2011 MACStats tables and figures include data and information for all Medicaid eligibility groups. However, the discussion at the front of each section has a particular focus on persons with disabilities—in part because these individuals account for a small portion of Medicaid enrollees but a substantial portion of the program's spending growth, a key issue for states and the federal government as they consider options for slowing that growth. The Commission will examine this population and others, including those dually eligible for Medicaid and Medicare, in greater depth in future reports to the Congress. In addition, future Commission work will examine CHIP enrollment and spending in greater depth.

MACStats

In this June 2011 *Report to the Congress: The Evolution of Managed Care in Medicaid,* MACStats is divided into four sections:

▷ Section 1: Trends in Medicaid Enrollment and Spending

▷ Section 2: Medicaid and CHIP Populations

▷ Section 3: Medicaid Managed Care

▷ Section 4: Technical Guide to the June 2011 MACStats

Following are some key points in the June 2011 MACStats, which include the fact that in many Medicaid program statistics, persons with disabling conditions may not be easy to identify. Although many individuals have complex health care needs or conditions that might be considered disabling (Tables 3A-5C), the term "disabled" in the Medicaid program generally refers to individuals under age 65 who qualify for federal Supplemental Security Income (SSI) benefits or meet similar criteria (Section 4 of MACStats).

Section 1: Trends in Medicaid Enrollment and Spending

▷ Individuals with disabilities account for a disproportionate share of Medicaid benefit spending growth (Table 2).

▷ Individuals age 65 and older account for about 60 percent of dual eligible enrollees (i.e., those enrolled in both Medicaid and Medicare) and dual eligible Medicaid benefit spending; younger dual eligibles account for the remaining 40 percent (Tables 6 and 7).

Section 2: Medicaid and CHIP Populations

▷ Medicaid/CHIP enrollees differ from individuals with other types of coverage, as well as from each other when subgroups of enrollees are examined, in terms of health status and the presence of certain health conditions (Tables 3A-5C).[1]

▷ Disabled and aged enrollees have per enrollee Medicaid benefit spending that is three to five times larger than that of other children and adults (Figure 4), with wide variation by state (Table 8).

▷ LTSS users account for a small share of Medicaid enrollees but a large share of Medicaid spending that includes both LTSS and acute care (Figures 5-7).

Section 3: Medicaid Managed Care

▷ Depending on the definition used, the percentage of Medicaid enrollees in managed care ranges from less than half to more than 70 percent (Table 9).

▷ Non-disabled children and adults under age 65 are more likely to be enrolled in managed care than persons with disabilities and individuals age 65 and older (Table 11).

---

[1] Health and other characteristics presented in Tables 3A-5C are for the Medicaid/CHIP population as a whole because the data source (the National Health Interview Survey) does not publish separate results for Medicaid and CHIP enrollees. The other tables and figures in Section 2 are specific to Medicaid.

MACStats

Section 4: Technical Guide to the June 2011 MACStats

There are several key issues to be aware of when interpreting the June 2011 MACStats. Section 4 provides a guide to these issues, which are briefly summarized here.

- **Sources of Variation in Medicaid and CHIP Numbers.** Data on Medicaid and CHIP enrollees and spending are available from a variety of sources. Each may produce unique insights into the programs and their enrollees' characteristics; however, the number of enrollees and program spending can vary across the different sources. Much of this is attributable to differences that are described in greater detail in Section 4, including the sources of data, the enrollment period examined, and the individuals included in the analyses.

- **Medicaid Statistics on Persons with Disabilities.** Individuals under age 65 who qualify for Medicaid on the basis of a disability are categorized in most Medicaid program statistics as disabled, rather than as children or adults. Conversely, there may be some individuals with disabilities—broadly defined—who are counted in the child and adult categories, if those individuals do not receive SSI benefits or meet similar criteria. Adults age 65 and older are included in the aged category regardless of disability status. As a result, there are many Medicaid enrollees who have physical or mental impairments that might be considered disabling but who are not counted as disabled in various program statistics.

- **MACPAC Adjustments to Spending Data.** The FY 2008 Medicaid benefit spending amounts reported in the June 2011 MACStats were calculated based on Medicaid Statistical Information System (MSIS) data that have been adjusted to match total benefit spending reported by states in CMS-64 data.[2] Although the CMS-64 provides a more complete accounting of spending and is preferred when examining state or federal totals, MSIS is the only data source that allows for analysis of benefit spending by eligibility group and other enrollee characteristics. The extent to which MSIS differs from the CMS-64 varies by state, meaning that a cross-state comparison of unadjusted MSIS amounts may not reflect true differences in benefit spending. By adjusting the MSIS data, we are attempting to provide comparable estimates of Medicaid benefit spending across states that can be analyzed by eligibility group and other enrollee characteristics. Other organizations, including the Office of the Actuary at CMS, the Kaiser Commission on Medicaid and the Uninsured, and the Urban Institute, use methodologies that are similar to MACPAC's but may differ in various ways. More on MACPAC's methodology is included in Section 4.

- **Sources of Variation in Medicaid Managed Care Numbers.** In MACStats and the managed care discussion in this Report, many of the statistics cited on managed care are from the *2009 Medicaid Managed Care Enrollment Report* published by CMS. However, the enrollment report does not provide information on characteristics of enrollees in managed care (e.g., basis of eligibility and demographics such as age, sex, and race/ethnicity) aside from dual eligibility status, nor their spending and non-managed care service use. As a result, we supplement statistics from the enrollment report with MSIS and CMS-64 data, which differ from each other in a variety of ways that are noted in Section 4.

---

[2] For a discussion of these data sources, see MACPAC, Improving Medicaid and CHIP Data for Policy Analysis and Program Accountability, in *Report to the Congress on Medicaid and CHIP: March 2011*. http://www.macpac.gov/reports/MACPAC_March2011_web.pdf.

MACStats

MAC Stats

SECTION

Trends in Medicaid Enrollment and Spending

Overall Medicaid spending growth is driven by growth in the number of people covered by Medicaid and in program spending per person. Both have grown at different rates over time, as illustrated in Figure 1. Sometimes this growth (or lack thereof) was driven by broad economic changes; at other times, trends in Medicaid enrollment and spending reflected changes in federal and state Medicaid policies.

For example, in the late 1970s and early 1980s, inflation levels were high economy-wide, causing rapid Medicaid spending growth while enrollment was flat. From the mid-1980s to the mid-1990s, numerous Medicaid-specific changes occurred, such as eligibility expansions and states' use of supplemental payments and alternative financing mechanisms. In the mid- to late 1990s, program growth was affected by federal Medicaid changes—primarily welfare reform, which delinked Medicaid eligibility for low-income families from the receipt of cash welfare assistance.[3] In the mid-2000s, enrollment growth slowed. Spending actually declined from FY 2005 to FY 2006, primarily because of the shift of dual eligibles' outpatient prescription drug spending from Medicaid to Medicare Part D.[4] In the early and late 2000s, the economic recessions spurred increased program enrollment and, thus, program spending.[5]

Total Medicaid spending can be measured in different ways, as can the number of program participants. In turn, these measurement differences can affect how much spending growth is attributed to the number of people covered versus program spending per person.

---

[3] For a discussion of growth from the program's beginnings through the late 1990s, see J. Klemm, Medicaid spending: A brief history, *Health Care Financing Review* 22 (Fall 2000): 105-112. https://www.cms.gov/HealthCareFinancingReview/Downloads/00fallpg105.pdf.

[4] J. Holahan et al., *Why did Medicaid spending decline in 2006? A detailed look at program spending and enrollment, 2000-2006* (Washington, DC: Kaiser Commission on Medicaid and the Uninsured, Issue Paper #7697, October 2007). http://www.kff.org/medicaid/upload/7697.pdf. .

[5] Holahan and A. Yemane, Enrollment is driving Medicaid costs—But two targets can yield savings, *Health Affairs* 28 (2009): 1453-1465.

MACStats

For example, Figure 2 shows three different ways to express Medicaid spending. First, Medicaid spending is shown in nominal, or current, dollars—that is, in the dollar amounts for each respective year. However, more items and services could be purchased for a dollar in 1975 than in 2008. There are two ways to adjust for this effect. One is to convert nominal historical spending to real, inflation-adjusted amounts based on *economy-wide* inflation. This is the approach commonly taken among organizations and researchers whose scope is not limited to health care, such as the Congressional Budget Office (CBO).[6] A second alternative, used by CMS, is to convert nominal historical Medicaid spending to real dollars using *health care* inflation,[7] which has generally exceeded economy-wide inflation. Using real dollars adjusted for health care inflation places Medicaid spending in the context of the overall U.S. health care system—recognizing that Medicaid faces the same cost pressures as other health care payers.

As shown in Figure 2, real historical Medicaid spending adjusted for health care inflation is higher than when adjusted for economy-wide inflation. This is because health care inflation has exceeded economy-wide inflation in most years.

To understand why the real historical Medicaid spending amounts shown in Figure 2 are higher when adjusted for health care inflation—and lower when adjusted for economy-wide inflation—it is helpful to consider the fact that inflation increases the dollar amount required to purchase the same amount of goods and services over time. As a result, to reproduce a purchase of goods and services in the health care sector in FY 1975 (or any year between FY 1975 and FY 2008) using FY 2008 dollars, the FY 2008 dollar amount must be larger than the original dollar amount to account for health care inflation. Since health care inflation generally exceeded economy-wide inflation over the period FY 1975 to FY 2008, an FY 2008 dollar amount that accounts only for economy-wide inflation—of which health care is just one component—would not be sufficient to reproduce that same health sector purchase.

Table 2 decomposes growth in Medicaid benefit spending[8] from FY 1975 to FY 2008 into two factors: the number of people served by Medicaid ("beneficiaries" or "recipients" as described in Section 4), and per beneficiary spending. According to this MACPAC analysis, growth in the number of beneficiaries is responsible for 68 percent of real (i.e., health care inflation-adjusted) Medicaid benefit spending growth from FY 1975 to FY 2008.[9] The remaining 32 percent is attributable to per beneficiary spending, which can reflect a number of factors, such as the changing breadth of Medicaid benefit packages, increased health care utilization or treatment intensity specific to

---

[6] For example, see: Congressional Budget Office (CBO), *The Long-Term Budget Outlook, June 2010 (revised August 2010)* (Washington, DC: CBO, 2010), http://www.cbo.gov/ftpdocs/115xx/ doc11579/06-30-LTBO.pdf; CBO, Appendix B in *The Long-Term Outlook for Health Care Spending* (Washington, DC: CBO, 2007), http://www.cbo.gov/ ftpdocs/87xx/doc8758/11-13-LT-Health.pdf; and CBO, Table 2 in *Medicaid Spending Growth and Options for Controlling Costs* (Washington, DC: CBO, 2006), http://www.cbo.gov/ftpdocs/73xx/doc7387/07-13-Medicaid.pdf..

[7] See, for example, Table 13.10 in CMS, *Health Care Financing Review 2010 Statistical Supplement*, 2010. https://www.cms.gov/MedicareMedicaidStatSupp/09_2010.asp

[8] Benefit spending excludes administration and the Vaccines for Children program. As described in Section 4, FY 2008 benefit spending amounts are from MSIS and have been adjusted to match totals reported by states in CMS-64 data. FY 1975 spending amounts do not need a similar adjustment because the data on which benefit spending were based in that year closely matched the CMS-64.

[9] Results can differ if using different years or eras. The period FY 1975 to FY 2008 is used here to examine factors driving growth over the Medicaid program's long history, rather than a particular time period (e.g., recent growth fueled by recessions in the early and late 2000s). Historical analyses of Medicaid spending often begin with FY 1975, after the program had stabilized following its initial startup growth.

Medicaid, and state and federal policies regarding provider payments, care management and other issues.[10]

The FY 1975–FY 2008 decomposition of growth by eligibility groups—aged, disabled, children, and adults—reveals that half of overall Medicaid benefit spending growth was attributable to enrollees with disabilities. This is driven mostly by enrollment growth for this population, which has outpaced all other groups (Table 2). Children accounted for approximately 21 percent of Medicaid spending growth between FY 1975 and FY 2008. Over that period, the aged and other adults each accounted for approximately 15 percent and 14 percent, respectively, of Medicaid benefit spending growth.

By FY 2008, the number of disabled beneficiaries had risen to 8.7 million, from 2.5 million in FY 1975. Although some of this increase is due to growth in the number of disabled individuals in the general population and the number of individuals receiving SSI benefits, some is due to federal Medicaid expansions since the 1980s that increased the number of persons with disabilities enrolled in the program, including home and community-based waivers and the Medicare Savings Programs (MSPs) under which state Medicaid programs pay all or some of low-income Medicare beneficiaries' Medicare premiums and cost sharing.[11]

Although children experienced the largest enrollment increase in absolute numbers, their annual growth rates were lower than those for the disabled. In addition, because the per recipient spending for children is low, it has a smaller impact on overall growth in Medicaid benefit spending.

---

[10] As noted in the text, the real Medicaid spending figures used in this calculation are adjusted for health care inflation. If the real Medicaid spending figures were instead adjusted for economy-wide inflation, the portion of growth attributable to per beneficiary spending would be higher— because health care inflation in excess of economy-wide inflation would be added to the list of explanatory factors such as the changing breadth of Medicaid benefit packages. For example, if the FY 1975 spending amounts were converted to real dollars using economy-wide inflation rather than health care inflation, only 40 percent of real Medicaid benefit spending growth would be attributable to growth in the number of beneficiaries, and per beneficiary spending would account for 60 percent of the growth.

[11] MSPs—the Qualified Medicare Beneficiary (QMB) Program, Specified Low-Income Medicare Beneficiary (SLMB) Program, and Qualifying Individual (QI) Program—are administered by state Medicaid programs; the amount of Medicare premiums and cost sharing (i.e., deductibles and coinsurance) paid varies by the type of MSP. See Social Security Administration, *Trends in the Social Security and Supplemental Security Income Disability Programs* (Baltimore, MD: SSA Publication No. 13-1183, August 2006): 29. http://www.socialsecurity.gov/policy/docs/chartbooks/disability_trends/trends.pdf.

FIGURE 1.   Medicaid Enrollment and Spending, FY 1966–FY 2010

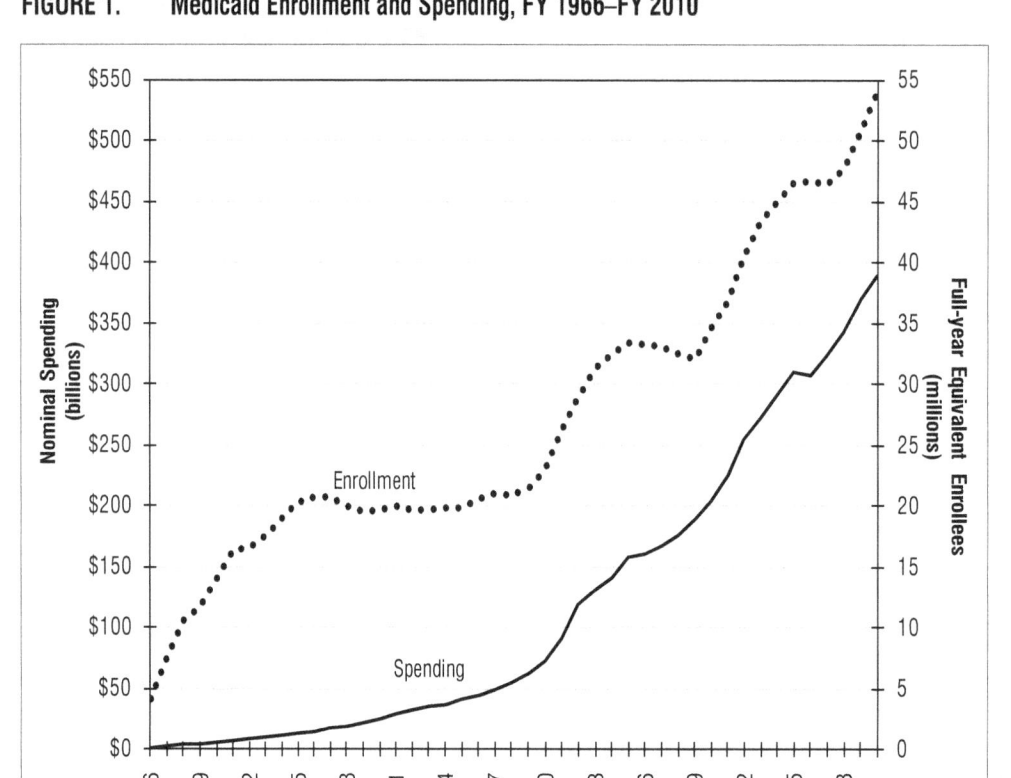

Notes: Data prior to FY 1977 have been adjusted to new fiscal year basis (Oct. 1 - Sep. 30); data for FY 2009 and FY 2010 are projected. Spending includes federal and state funds for benefits and administration; excludes the Vaccines for Children program; may differ from amounts published elsewhere due to slight differences in the timing of data and the treatment of certain adjustments. Enrollment counts are full-year equivalents and have been estimated from counts of persons served for fiscal years prior to FY 1990 (see Section 4 of MACStats for a discussion of how enrollees are counted). Excludes Medicaid-expansion CHIP.

Source: Data compilation provided to MACPAC by Centers for Medicare & Medicaid Services, Office of the Actuary, May 2011

FIGURE 2. **Medicaid Spending in Nominal and Real Dollars, FY 1975–FY 2008**

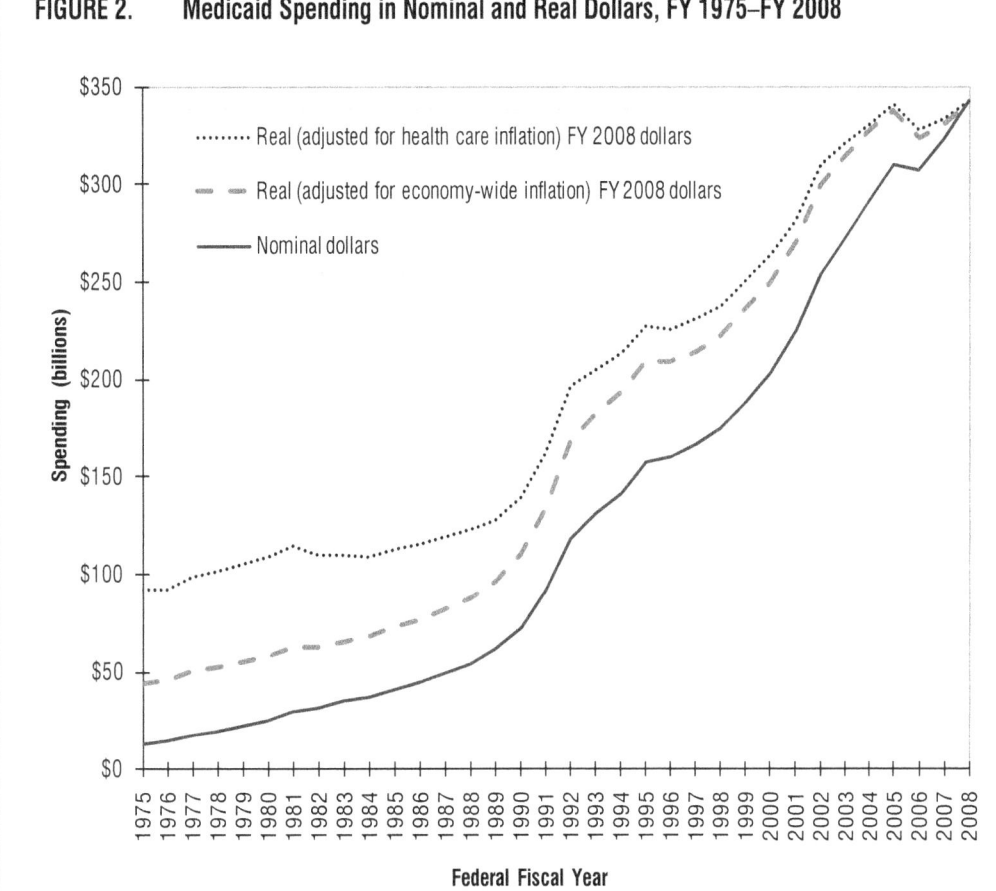

Notes: Includes benefits and administrative spending. The bottom line in the figure shows actual (nominal) spending. The middle line transforms nominal Medicaid spending to real FY 2008 dollars by adjusting for economy-wide inflation, using the Gross Domestic Product (GDP) price deflator. The top line also shows real FY 2008 dollars, but based on inflation for health care in particular. Real historical Medicaid spending adjusted for health care inflation is higher than when adjusted for economy-wide inflation, which reflects the long history of health care inflation in excess of economy-wide inflation. The drop in spending for FY 2006, compared to FY 2005, is partly the result of the implementation of Medicare Part D.

Sources: Nominal Medicaid spending from Figure 1; real spending based on MACPAC analysis of nominal spending and quarterly National Income and Product Account (NIPA) historical tables, Quarter 1 of 2011

SECTION 1

MACStats

TABLE 1. Number of Medicaid Persons Served (Beneficiaries or Recipients), by Eligibility Group, FY 1975–FY 2008 (thousands)

Year	Total	Children	Adults	Disabled	Aged	Unknown
1975	22,007	9,598	4,529	2,464	3,615	1,801
1976	22,815	9,924	4,773	2,669	3,612	1,837
1977	22,832	9,651	4,785	2,802	3,636	1,958
1978	21,965	9,376	4,643	2,718	3,376	1,852
1979	21,520	9,106	4,570	2,753	3,364	1,727
1980	21,605	9,333	4,877	2,911	3,440	1,044
1981	21,980	9,581	5,187	3,079	3,367	766
1982	21,603	9,563	5,356	2,891	3,240	553
1983	21,554	9,535	5,592	2,921	3,372	134
1984	21,607	9,684	5,600	2,913	3,238	172
1985	21,814	9,757	5,518	3,012	3,061	466
1986	22,515	10,029	5,647	3,182	3,140	517
1987	23,109	10,168	5,599	3,381	3,224	737
1988	22,907	10,037	5,503	3,487	3,159	721
1989	23,511	10,318	5,717	3,590	3,132	754
1990	25,255	11,220	6,010	3,718	3,202	1,105
1991	27,967	12,855	6,703	4,033	3,341	1,035
1992	31,150	15,200	7,040	4,487	3,749	674
1993	33,432	16,285	7,505	5,016	3,863	763
1994	35,053	17,194	7,586	5,458	4,035	780
1995	36,282	17,164	7,604	5,858	4,119	1,537
1996	36,118	16,739	7,127	6,221	4,285	1,746
1997	34,872	15,791	6,803	6,129	3,955	2,195
1998	40,096	18,969	7,895	6,637	3,964	2,631
1999	39,748	18,233	7,446	6,690	3,698	3,682
2000	41,212	18,528	8,538	6,688	3,640	3,817
2001	45,164	20,181	9,707	7,114	3,812	4,349
2002	46,839	21,487	10,847	7,182	3,789	3,534
2003	50,716	23,742	11,530	7,664	4,041	3,739
2004	54,250	25,415	12,325	8,123	4,349	4,037
2005	56,276	25,979	12,431	8,205	4,395	5,266
2006	56,264	26,358	12,495	8,334	4,374	4,703
2007	55,210	26,061	12,264	8,423	4,044	4,418
2008[1]	56,962	26,479	12,739	8,685	4,147	4,912

Notes: Beneficiaries are shown here because they provide the only historical time series data directly available prior to FY 1990. Most current analyses of individuals in Medicaid reflect enrollees. For additional discussion, see Section 4 of MACStats. The increase in FY 1998 reflects a change in how Medicaid beneficiaries are counted. Beginning in FY 1998, a Medicaid-eligible person who, during the year, received only coverage for managed care benefits was included in this series as a beneficiary. Excludes Medicaid-expansion CHIP children. Children and non-aged adults who qualify for Medicaid on the basis of a disability are included in the disabled category. Generally, individuals whose eligibility group is unknown are persons who were enrolled in the prior year but had a Medicaid claim paid in the current year.

1 This table shows the number of beneficiaries. See Table 6 for the number of Medicaid enrollees in FY 2008 data from CMS.

Sources: For FY 1999 to FY 2008: MACPAC analysis of Medicaid Statistical Information System (MSIS) as of May 2011. For FY 1975 to FY 1998: Centers for Medicare & Medicaid Services (CMS) *Medicare & Medicaid Statistical Supplement, 2010 edition*, Table 13.4

TABLE 2. Components of Growth in Real Medicaid Benefit Spending, FY 1975–FY 2008

	FY 1975 (in FY 2008 dollars)	FY 2008	Annual Growth Rate	Relative Contribution to Real Spending Growth, FY 1975 to FY 2008
All Eligibility Groups				
Spending per beneficiary	$4,234	$6,504[1]	1.3%	32.2%
Number of beneficiaries (millions)	20.2	52.1	2.9%	67.8%
Total benefit spending (millions)	**$85,549**	**$338,552**	**4.3%**	**100.0%**
Children				
Spending per beneficiary	$1,658	$2,571[1]	1.3%	4.9%
Number of beneficiaries (millions)	9.6	26.5	3.1%	15.7%
Total benefit spending (millions)	**$15,914**	**$68,080**	**4.5%**	**20.6%**
Adults				
Spending per beneficiary	$3,315	$3,887[1]	0.5%	1.2%
Number of beneficiaries (millions)	4.5	12.7	3.2%	12.5%
Total benefit spending (millions)	**$15,012**	**$49,512**	**3.7%**	**13.6%**
Disabled				
Spending per beneficiary	$9,292	$17,332[1]	1.9%	12.9%
Number of beneficiaries (millions)	2.5	8.7	3.9%	37.6%
Total benefit spending (millions)	**$22,896**	**$150,531**	**5.9%**	**50.4%**
Aged				
Spending per beneficiary	$8,776	$16,984[1]	2.0%	13.2%
Number of beneficiaries (millions)	3.6	4.1	0.4%	2.1%
Total benefit spending (millions)	**$31,727**	**$70,429**	**2.4%**	**15.3%**

Notes: Beneficiaries are shown here because they provide the only historical time series data available prior to FY 1990. Most current analyses of individuals in Medicaid reflect enrollees, as shown in Table 6. For additional discussion of the definitions of enrollees and beneficiaries, see Section 4 of MACStats.

Dollar amounts were adjusted for inflation using the Gross Domestic Product (GDP) price deflator for health care (see text for additional discussion). In this table, real Medicaid spending growth is attributed to either spending per beneficiary or number of beneficiaries, where the interaction of the two factors is allocated according to the shares separately attributable to spending per beneficiary and the number of beneficiaries.

Children and non-aged adults who qualify for Medicaid on the basis of a disability are included in the disabled category.

The number of beneficiaries excludes individuals whose basis of Medicaid eligibility is unknown. In this analysis, FY 1975 benefit spending for these individuals was allocated proportionally to the four eligibility groups in the table. FY 2008 benefit spending reflects MSIS data that have been adjusted to match CMS-64 totals; see Section 4 of MACStats for a discussion of the methodology used.

Results can differ if using different years or eras. The period FY 1975 to FY 2008 is used here to examine factors driving growth over the Medicaid program's long history, rather than a particular time period (e.g., recent growth fueled by recessions in the early and late 2000s).

1 Benefit spending per beneficiary shown here differs from the FY 2008 benefit spending per full-year equivalent enrollee shown in Table 8.

Sources: MACPAC analysis using data from CMS, 2010 Medicare and Medicaid Statistical Supplement (FY 1975), and from Medicaid Statistical Information System (MSIS) and CMS-64 net financial management report data (FY 2008)

MACStats

SECTION 2

Medicaid and CHIP Populations

This section of MACStats shows how Medicaid and CHIP enrollees differ from individuals with other types of coverage in terms of their general health, disability and work status, their need for assistance with activities of daily living (ADLs), and other characteristics (Tables 3A-5C). It also indicates that Medicaid populations—for example, low-income non-disabled children and adults, persons with disabilities, and individuals age 65 and older—differ markedly from each other in their characteristics, service use, and spending (shown throughout Section 2).

Health and Other Characteristics of Medicaid/CHIP Populations (Tables 3A-5C)

Every year, thousands of non-institutionalized[12] Americans are interviewed about their health insurance and health status for the National Health Interview Survey (NHIS), which is the source of data for Tables 3A through 5C. The NHIS is an annual face-to-face household survey of civilian non-institutionalized persons designed to monitor the health of the U.S. population through the collection of information on a broad range of health topics.[13] Administered by the National Center for Health Statistics (NCHS) within the Centers for Disease Control and Prevention (CDC), the NHIS consists of a nationally representative sample from approximately 35,000 households containing about 87,500 people.[14] Tables 3A through 5C are based on NHIS data, pooling the years 2007 through 2009.[15] Although there are other federal surveys, NHIS is used here because it is

---

[12] Although the discussion below generally omits the term "non-institutionalized" for brevity, all estimates exclude individuals living in nursing homes and other institutional settings.

[13] Centers for Disease Control and Prevention (CDC), About the National Health Interview Survey, last modified April 18, 2011. http://www.cdc.gov/nchs/nhis/about_nhis.htm.

[14] The annual NHIS questionnaire consists of three major components—the Family Core, the Sample Adult Core, and the Sample Child Core. The Family Core collects information for all family members regarding household composition, socio-demographic characteristics, along with basic indicators of health status, activity limitation, and health insurance. The Sample Adult and Sample Child Cores obtain additional information on the health of one randomly selected adult and child in the family.

[15] Data were pooled to yield sufficiently large samples to produce reliable subgroup estimates and to increase the capacity to detect meaningful differences between subgroups and insurance categories.

MACStats

SECTION 2

MACStats

generally considered to be one of the best surveys for health insurance coverage estimates, and it captures detailed information on individuals' health status.[16]

Tables 3A-C provide estimates of children age 0-18, Tables 4A-C of adults age 19-64, and Tables 5A-C of adults age 65 and older. Each age group's tables display the following:

- Health insurance coverage and demographics: Tables 3A, 4A, and 5A;

- Health: Tables 3B, 4B, and 5B; and

- Use of health care: Tables 3C, 4C, and 5C.

All of these tables are broken into two parts—first comparing Medicaid/CHIP enrollees in that age group to individuals with other sources of health insurance, then comparing subgroups of Medicaid/CHIP enrollees with each other.[17]

Children Under Age 19

Table 3A, which focuses on children's health insurance status and demographics, shows that 32.1 percent of children were Medicaid/CHIP enrollees, while 57.6 percent of children were in private coverage and 9.1 percent were uninsured. The table then provides estimates of how those children's characteristics differ, depending on their source of health insurance, with an asterisk noting where those differences from Medicaid/CHIP children are statistically significant. For example, Medicaid/CHIP children are more likely to be Hispanic (32.9 percent) than privately insured children (12.2 percent) and less likely to be Hispanic than uninsured children (38.6 percent);

Medicaid/CHIP children are more likely to be non-Hispanic black (24.6 percent) than privately insured (9.5 percent) or uninsured children (10.6 percent).

Table 3B, which focuses on children's health, shows that Medicaid/CHIP children are more likely than privately insured or uninsured children to be in fair or poor health and to have certain impairments and health conditions (e.g., ADHD/ADD, asthma). Table 3C, which focuses on children's health care use, shows that Medicaid/CHIP children were more likely to have had a visit to the emergency room in the past year, and to have been regularly taking prescription medications for at least three months.

The right-hand portion of Tables 3A-C groups the Medicaid/CHIP enrollees under age 19 into mutually exclusive categories:

- Children who receive Supplemental Security Income (SSI) benefits and are therefore disabled under that program's definition;[18]

- Children who do not receive SSI but who are classified as children with special health care needs (CSHCN); and

- Children who neither receive SSI nor are considered CSHCN.

CSHCN are defined by the Maternal and Child Health Bureau (MCHB) within the Health Resources and Services Administration (HRSA) as a group of children who "have or are at increased risk for a chronic physical, developmental, behavioral, or emotional condition and who also require health and related services of a type or amount beyond that required by children

---

[16] G. Kenney and V. Lynch, Monitoring children's health insurance coverage under CHIPRA using federal surveys, in *Databases for estimating health insurance coverage for children: A workshop summary*, edited by T. Plewes (Washington, DC: The National Academies Press, 2010): 72. http://www.nap.edu/catalog/13024.html.

[17] Health and other characteristics presented in Tables 3A-5C are for the Medicaid/CHIP population as a whole because the data source (the National Health Interview Survey) does not publish separate results for Medicaid and CHIP enrollees.

[18] For a discussion of disability as determined under the SSI program, see the discussion of Medicaid eligibility for persons with disabilities in MACStats Section 4.

SECTION 2

generally."[19] This definition, which is used by all states for policy and program planning purposes for CSHCN, is a broad classification that encompasses children with disabilities and also children with chronic conditions (e.g., asthma, juvenile diabetes, sickle cell anemia) that range from mild to severe. It includes children who are "at risk" of these conditions and those who have been diagnosed, as well as children who require "related services" not traditionally considered health services (for example, social and home care services, school and developmental programs).

Very few children have conditions severe enough and family incomes so low as to qualify for SSI (see Section 4). Therefore, CSHCN designation is intended to capture a broader group of children with chronic health conditions. Many researchers use the MCHB definition for CSHCN, although they may not include the at-risk population in their analyses. MACPAC analyses of CSHCN in this Report may not fully include the at-risk population. Based on an approach developed by researchers,[20] children with special health care needs are identified in MACStats as those who have at least one of five broad symptoms of a chronic health problem as a result of a health condition lasting at least 12 months. By this definition, a CSHCN:

- is limited or prevented in his or her ability to do things most children of the same age can do;

- needs or uses medications prescribed by a doctor (other than vitamins);

- needs or uses specialized therapies such as physical, occupational, or speech therapy;

- has above-routine need or use of medical, mental health, or education services; or

- needs or receives treatment or counseling for an emotional, behavioral, or developmental problem.[21]

It should be noted that CSHCN can vary substantially in their health status and use of health care services. A CSHCN could be a child with intensive health care needs and high health care expenses who has severe functional limitations (e.g., spina bifida, cerebral palsy, paralysis) and would qualify for SSI if his or her family income were low enough.[22] On the other hand, a CSHCN could also be a child who has asthma, attention deficit disorder, or depression that is well managed through the use of prescription medications. Regardless of whether functional limitations are mild, moderate or severe, however, CSHCN share a heightened need for health care services in order to maintain their health and to be able to function appropriately for their age.

As described earlier, many health and demographic characteristics of children enrolled in Medicaid/CHIP differ significantly from children with other coverage. In addition, among the children enrolled

[19] M. McPherson et al., A new definition of children with special health care needs, *Pediatrics* 102 (1998): 137-140.

[20] C. Bethell et al., Identifying children with special health needs: Development and evaluation of a short screening instrument, *Ambulatory Pediatrics* 2 (2002): 38-48.

[21] Since the NHIS does not explicitly include the standard CSHCN screening questions, this analysis uses an adaptation developed by Christine Coyer of the Urban Institute for the 2007-2009 NHIS based on an operationalization of the CSHCN screener for the 1999-2000 NHIS (Davidoff, A. Identifying children with special health care needs in the National Health Interview Survey: A new resource for policy analysis, *Health Services Research*, 39 (2004): 53-72). While the method used in this edition of MACStats attempts to replicate the standard CSHCN screener as much as possible, there are other ways to operationalize the CSHCN definition using the NHIS.

[22] For a child to be eligible for SSI, one of the criteria is that the child has a medically determinable physical or mental impairment(s) that results in marked and severe functional limitations and generally is expected to last 12 months or result in death. Thus, children who are receiving SSI should meet the criteria for being a child with special health care needs (CSHCN); however, some do not. While we do not have enough information to assess the reasons that these Medicaid/CHIP children who are reported to have SSI did not meet the criteria for CSHCN, it could be because (1) the parent erroneously reported the child's receipt of SSI in the survey, or (2) the parent correctly reported SSI but neglected to report the child's health information related to his/her eligibility for SSI and thus classification as a CSHCN.

MACStats

SECTION 2

MACStats

in Medicaid/CHIP, the three subgroups identified often vary significantly from Medicaid/CHIP children overall:

▷ **Significant differences in general health exist among children enrolled in Medicaid/CHIP.** As shown in the right-hand portion of Table 3B, among children enrolled in Medicaid/CHIP, 18.5 percent of those receiving SSI are in fair or poor health, compared to 11.4 percent for non-SSI CSHCN and 1.0 percent for children who are neither SSI nor CSHCN.[23]

▷ **Incidence of specific health conditions varies among children enrolled in Medicaid/CHIP.** As shown in the right-hand portion of Table 3B, the incidence of ADHD/ADD among Medicaid-CHIP enrolled children is 39.0 percent for SSI children, 39.4 percent for non-SSI CSHCN, and 1.9 percent for children who are neither SSI nor CSHCN. The incidence of asthma reported by SSI children was 30.1 percent, compared to 40.8 percent for non-SSI CSHCN and 10.7 percent for children who are neither SSI nor CSHCN.

▷ **Significant differences in use of recent care exist among children enrolled in Medicaid/CHIP.** As shown in the right-hand portion of Table 3C, SSI children and non-SSI CSHCN are each nearly twice as likely to visit health care providers four or more times within a year than Medicaid/CHIP children who are neither SSI nor CSHCN.

Adults Age 19-64

According to the NHIS estimates shown in Table 4A, 8.4 percent of non-institutionalized adults age 19-64 were enrolled in Medicaid or CHIP.[24] The Medicaid/CHIP enrollees in this age group tend to be in much worse health than those enrolled in private coverage or the uninsured, but in better health than those enrolled in Medicare.

Dual eligibles are individuals who are enrolled in both Medicaid and Medicare.[25] For 19-64-year-olds, dual eligibles are low-income individuals who are eligible for Medicare on the basis of a disability and for Medicaid on a basis that may or may not include disability.[26] Table 4A shows that Medicaid/CHIP enrollees in this age group, 12.4 percent also were enrolled in Medicare; conversely, of the Medicare enrollees in this age group, 31.0 percent also were enrolled in Medicaid.

The right-hand portion of Tables 4A-C groups the 19-64-year-old Medicaid/CHIP enrollees into three mutually exclusive categories:

▷ Dual eligibles;

▷ Medicaid enrollees receiving SSI who are not dual eligibles; and

▷ Medicaid/CHIP enrollees who are neither SSI nor Medicare enrollees.

The right-hand portions of Tables 4A-C illustrate how these groups of individuals vary significantly from 19-64-year-old Medicaid/CHIP enrollees overall:

---

[23] Although this particular statistical significance testing is not displayed in Table 3B, all of these estimates are significantly different from one another.

[24] Federal surveys such as NHIS do not publish separate results for Medicaid and CHIP enrollment. CHIP enrollment of adults is small, totaling less than 350,000 ever enrolled during FY 2010 (Table 3, March 2011 MACStats).

[25] Enrollment in CHIP-financed coverage is prohibited for those with other coverage, such as Medicare.

[26] Most dual eligibles under age 65 have obtained their Medicare coverage after a two-year waiting period following their initial receipt of Social Security Disability Insurance (SSDI) benefits. During the two-year waiting period and beyond, SSDI beneficiaries may have incomes low enough to qualify for SSI benefits and therefore Medicaid; they may also qualify for Medicaid via other pathways (e.g., as a low-income parent or an individual with high medical expenses who "spends down" to a Medicaid income eligibility level). For information on SSI and SSDI, see the discussion of Medicaid eligibility for persons with disabilities in Section 4.

Significant differences in general health exist among 19-64-year-olds enrolled in Medicaid/CHIP. Table 4B shows that dual eligibles and the non-dual SSI beneficiaries report fair or poor health (62.9 percent and 57.9 percent, respectively)[27] at much higher rates than non-SSI, non-dual enrollees (21.3 percent).

Among 19-64-year-olds enrolled in Medicaid/CHIP, incidence of specific health conditions is highest for persons with disabilities. Table 4B also shows that dual eligibles and non-dual SSI beneficiaries were more likely to report the presence of chronic conditions such as heart disease, diabetes, depression, chronic bronchitis and arthritis than the overall Medicaid/CHIP enrollees in this age group.

Table 4C shows that among 19-64-year-olds enrolled in Medicaid/CHIP, persons with disabilities have higher use of recent care. Dual eligibles and non-dual SSI beneficiaries also made more visits to health care providers within a year and were more likely to receive home care within the past year than 19-64-year-old Medicaid/CHIP enrollees overall, as shown in Table 4C.

Adults Age 65 and Older

According to the NHIS estimates shown in Table 5A, 7.3 percent of non-institutionalized adults age 65 and older were enrolled in Medicaid.[28] Medicare covered 95.2 percent of those aged 65 and older.

Table 5A also shows that of Medicaid enrollees age 65 and older, 91.0 percent were dual eligibles.[29] Conversely, of the Medicare enrollees in this age group, 7.0 percent also were enrolled in Medicaid.

The right-hand portion of Tables 5A-C groups the Medicaid enrollees age 65 and older into two mutually exclusive categories:

- Those with a functional limitation; and
- Those without a functional limitation.

Individuals with a functional limitation are those who reported any degree of difficulty—ranging from "only a little difficult" to "can't do at all"—doing any of a dozen activities[30] by themselves and without special equipment. It should be noted that individuals with functional limitations can vary substantially in their health needs—from being bedridden in one's home[31] to being relatively healthy but responding that walking a quarter of a mile is "only a little difficult." The right-hand portion of Tables 5A-C illustrates how these two groups of individuals vary significantly from aged Medicaid/CHIP enrollees overall. However, because more than three-quarters of aged Medicaid enrollees have functional limitations, those with functional limitations drive the overall characteristics of aged enrollees, and thus do not show significant differences from the total as often as those with no functional limitations.

---

[27] Although this particular statistical significance testing is not displayed in Table 4B, these two estimates are significantly different from the estimate for non-dual SSI beneficiaries (21.3 percent).

[28] Even though survey estimates are generally not published separately for Medicaid and CHIP, CHIP is not included in this portion of the NHIS estimates because its occurrence among those aged 65 and older would be rare. Enrollment in CHIP-financed coverage is prohibited for those with other coverage, such as Medicare, and 95 percent of those 65 and older have Medicare.

[29] Nearly all individuals are entitled to Medicare coverage upon turning 65; as with Medicare enrollees under age 65, they may have incomes low enough or medical expenses high enough to also qualify for Medicaid.

[30] The activities asked about in the survey are the following: walk a quarter of a mile, walk up 10 steps without resting, stand or be on your feet for about two hours, sit for about two hours, stoop or kneel, reach up over your head, use your fingers to grasp or handle small objects, lift or carry something as heavy as 10 pounds, push or pull large objects like a living room chair, go out to do things like shopping, participate in social activities such as visiting friends, or do things to relax at home such as reading or watching TV.

[31] Individuals in institutions such as nursing homes are not interviewed in the NHIS.

MACStats

SECTION 2

TABLE 3A. Health Insurance and Demographic Characteristics of Non-institutionalized Individuals Age 0-18 by Source of Health Insurance, 2007–2009

	All Children	Selected Sources of Insurance[1]			Medicaid/CHIP children	Medicaid/CHIP[2]		
		Medicaid/CHIP[2]	Private[3]	Uninsured[4]		SSI	Non-SSI CSHCN[5]	Neither SSI nor CSHCN
Health Insurance Coverage		**32.1%**	57.6%	9.1%	**100.0%**	3.0%	17.9%	79.1%
Age (categories sum to 100%)								
0-5	32.2%*	**39.0%**	29.5%*	24.8%*	**39.0%**	16.7%*	24.5%*	43.2%*
6-11	30.6	**30.9**	30.7	29.2	**30.9**	34.6	38.1*	29.2
12-18	37.2*	**30.0**	39.8*	46.1*	**30.0**	48.7*	37.4*	27.6*
Gender (categories sum to 100%)								
Male	51.2%	**51.4%**	50.9%	50.9%	**51.4%**	62.9%*	60.0%*	49.0%*
Female	48.8	**48.6**	49.1	49.1	**48.6**	37.1*	40.0*	51.0*
Race (categories sum to 100%)								
Hispanic	21.4%*	**32.9%**	12.2%*	38.6%*	**32.9%**	23.8%*	21.5%*	35.8%*
White, non-Hispanic	56.2*	**35.0**	70.4*	42.9*	**35.0**	34.3	44.8*	32.9
Black, non-Hispanic	14.6*	**24.6**	9.5*	10.6*	**24.6**	36.5*	25.2	24.0
Other and multiple races, non-Hispanic	7.8	**7.5**	7.9	7.9	**7.5**	5.4	8.5	7.3
Health insurance								
Medicaid/CHIP	32.1%*	**100.0%**	2.4%*	–	**100.0%**	100.0%	100.0%	100.0%
Private	57.6*	**4.3**	100.0*	–	**4.3**	11.5*	6.3*	3.6

See Table 3C for sources and notes.

MACStats

SECTION 2

MACStats

TABLE 3B. Health Characteristics of Non-institutionalized Individuals Age 0-18 by Source of Health Insurance, 2007–2009

	All Children	Selected Sources of Insurance[1]			Medicaid/CHIP[2]			
		Medicaid/ CHIP[2]	Private[3]	Uninsured[4]	Medicaid/ CHIP children	SSI	Non-SSI CSHCN[5]	Neither SSI nor CSHCN
Children with disabilities or with special health care needs								
Receives supplemental security income (SSI)	1.2%*	**3.0%**	0.4%*	0.3%	**3.0%**	100.0%*	—	—
Children with special health care needs (CSHCN)[5]	14.8*	**20.3**	12.7*	11.3	**20.3**	79.7*[6]	100.0*	—
Current health status (categories sum to 100%)								
Excellent or very good	82.8%*	**72.7%**	89.2%*	76.9%*	**72.7%**	42.3%*	53.9%*	78.1%*
Good	15.4*	**23.9**	10.0*	20.9*	**23.9**	39.3*	34.7*	20.9*
Fair or poor	1.8*	**3.4**	0.8*	2.2*	**3.4**	18.5*	11.4*	1.0*
Impairments								
Impairment requiring special equipment	1.0%*	**1.5%**	1.0%*	0.3%*	**1.5%**	11.7%*	4.9%*	0.3%*
Impairment limits ability to crawl, walk, run, play[7]	1.8*	**2.5**	1.5*	1.4*	**2.5**	19.7*	8.2*	0.6*
Impairment lasted, or expected to last 12+ months[8]	1.6*	**2.3**	1.3*	1.3*	**2.3**	19.6*	7.7*	0.4*
Specific health conditions								
Ever told child has:								
ADHD/ADD[8]	7.5%*	**10.7%**	6.3%*	5.2%*	**10.7%**	39.0%*	39.4%*	1.9%*
Asthma	13.6*	**16.6**	12.7*	9.9*	**16.6**	30.1*	40.8*	10.7*
Autism[7]	0.8*	**1.1**	0.7*	†	**1.1**	10.2*	4.2*	†
Cerebral palsy[7]	0.7	**0.8**	0.8	0.6	**0.8**	6.8*	1.7*	0.3
Congenital heart disease	1.3	**1.5**	1.2	0.9*	**1.5**	5.1*	5.1*	0.6
Diabetes	0.2	**0.3**	0.2	†	**0.3**	†	1.1*	0.1
Down syndrome[7]	0.1	**0.2**	0.1	†	**0.2**	2.2*	0.8*	†
Mental retardation[7]	0.6*	**1.2**	0.3*	†	**1.2**	13.6*	4.4*	0.0
Other developmental delay[7]	4.0*	**5.8**	3.4*	2.7*	**5.8**	43.9*	21.8*	0.8
Sickle cell anemia[7]	0.2	**0.3**	0.1*	†	**0.3**	1.6	0.8*	0.1

See Table 3C for sources and notes.

TABLE 3C. Use of Care by Non-institutionalized Individuals Age 0-18 by Source of Health Insurance, 2007–2009

	All Children	Selected Sources of Insurance[1]			Medicaid/ CHIP children	Medicaid/CHIP[2]		
		Medicaid/ CHIP[2]	Private[3]	Uninsured[4]		SSI	Non-SSI CSHCN[5]	Neither SSI nor CSHCN
Received well-child check-up in past 12 months[7]	75.8%*	78.9%	78.5%	46.1%*	78.9%	83.0%	83.3%*	77.7%
Regularly taking prescription drug(s) for 3+ months[8]	12.8*	15.1	12.9*	5.8*	15.1	51.3*	52.9*	5.0*
Number of times saw a doctor or other health professional in past 12 months (categories sum to 100%)								
None	11.3%*	9.3%	8.6%	35.2%*	9.3%	6.1%	4.4%*	10.5%
1	21.4*	19.6	21.9*	23.6*	19.6	17.8	8.5*	22.1*
2-3	35.9	35.2	37.8*	26.3*	35.2	21.9*	27.3*	37.4*
4+	31.3*	36.0	31.7*	14.8*	36.0	54.2*	59.8*	30.0*
Number of emergency room visits in past 12 months (categories sum to 100%)								
None	79.3%*	71.6%	83.0%*	82.2%*	71.6%	61.1%*	59.9%	74.7%*
1	13.7*	17.0	12.1*	11.5*	17.0	23.1	20.8*	15.9
2-3	5.7*	8.7	4.3*	5.1*	8.7	7.7	13.3*	7.7
4+	1.3*	2.7	0.6*	1.2*	2.7	8.0*	5.9*	1.7*

Notes: Health insurance coverage is defined at the time of the survey. Totals of health insurance coverage may sum to more than 100% because individuals may have multiple sources of coverage. Responses to recent care questions are based on the previous 12 months, during which time the individual may have had different coverage than that shown in the table. In order to focus on a consistent sample across the measures included in this table, the tabulations reported here are based on the NHIS sample child/adult weights. Somewhat different estimates might be obtained using the broader person file weights for the subset of variables that are available for all persons in the household. This analysis provides conservative estimates of statistical significance; it does not take into account subgroups' non-independence by incorporating the covariance.

† Estimates with a relative standard error of greater than 50% are indicated with a dagger and are not shown.

* Difference from Medicaid/CHIP is statistically significant at the 95 percent confidence level.

– Quantity zero; amounts shown as 0.0 round to less than 0.1 in this table.

[1] Not separately shown are the estimates of children covered by Medicare (0.3%, generally children with end-stage renal disease, ESRD), any type of military health plan (VA, TRICARE, and CHAMP-VA), or other government programs.

[2] Medicaid/CHIP health insurance coverage also includes persons covered by other state-sponsored health plans.

[3] Private health insurance coverage excludes plans that paid for only one type of service, such as accidents or dental care.

[4] A person was defined as uninsured if he/she did not have any private health insurance, Medicaid, CHIP, Medicare, state-sponsored or other government-sponsored health plans, or military plan. A person was also defined as uninsured if he/she had only Indian Health Service (IHS) coverage or had only a private plan that paid for one type of service, such as accidents or dental care.

[5] A standard screener has been developed by researchers (Bethell et al., 2002) to identify children with special health care needs (CSHCN) as those who have at least one of five broad symptoms of a chronic health problem (e.g., needs or uses prescription medications) as a result of a health condition(s) lasting at least 12 months. Since the NHIS does not explicitly include the standard CSHCN screener, this analysis adapted Davidoff's (2004) methodology for identifying CSHCN which was developed for the 1999-2000 NHIS, to the 2007-2009 NHIS. While this method attempts to replicate the standard CSHCN screener as much as possible on the NHIS, there are other ways of operationalizing the CSHCN definition on the NHIS.

[6] For a child to be eligible for SSI, one of the criteria is that the child has a medically determinable physical or mental impairment(s) that result in marked and severe functional limitations and generally is expected to last at least 12 months or result in death. Thus, children who are eligible for SSI should meet the criteria for being a child with special health care needs (CSHCN); however, some do not. While we do not have enough information to assess the reasons that these Medicaid/CHIP children who are reported to have SSI did not meet the criteria for CSHCN, it could be because (1) the parents erroneously reported the child's receipt of SSI in the survey, or (2) the parents neglected to report in the survey the child's health information related to his/her eligibility for SSI and thus as a CSHCN

[7] Question only asked for children age 0 to 17.

[8] Question only asked for children age 2 to 17.

Source: Urban Institute analysis of the National Health Interview Survey (NHIS) for MACPAC; the estimates for 2007-2009 are based on household interviews of a sample of the civilian non-institutionalized population

MACStats

SECTION 2

MACStats

TABLE 4A. Health Insurance and Demographic Characteristics of Non-institutionalized Individuals Age 19-64 by Source of Health Insurance, 2007–2009

	All Non-aged Adults	Selected Sources of Insurance[1]				Medicaid/CHIP non-aged adults	Medicaid/CHIP[2]		
		Medicaid/CHIP[2]	Private[3]	Medicare	Uninsured[4]		Medicare (duals)	Non-dual SSI	Neither SSI nor Medicare
Health Insurance Coverage		8.4%	67.5%	3.4%	20.4%	100.0%	12.4%	16.0%	71.6%
Age (categories sum to 100%)									
19-24	13.5%*	17.8%	11.0%*	1.7%*	20.5%*	17.8%	1.4%*	9.8%*	22.6%*
25-44	44.4*	47.4	43.3*	23.3*	50.4*	47.4	34.4*	38.7*	51.7*
45-54	23.8*	19.4	25.9*	28.0*	18.3	19.4	30.4*	26.3*	15.8*
55-64	18.3*	15.4	19.7*	47.0*	10.8*	15.4	33.8*	25.2*	9.9*
Gender (categories sum to 100%)									
Male	49.3%*	33.7%	49.1%*	50.2%*	55.1%*	33.7%	44.0%*	38.6%*	30.7%*
Female	50.7*	66.3	50.9*	49.8*	44.9*	66.3	56.0*	61.4*	69.3*
Race (categories sum to 100%)									
Hispanic	14.8%*	22.0%	9.6%*	8.4%*	30.2%*	22.0%	9.0%*	15.0%*	25.9%*
White, non-Hispanic	66.4*	48.0	73.9*	67.9*	49.5	48.0	64.2*	52.1	44.3*
Black, non-Hispanic	12.1*	23.4	9.9*	18.4*	13.7*	23.4	20.6	27.6	22.8
Other and multiple races, non-Hispanic	6.7	6.6	6.7	5.3*	6.6	6.6	6.2	5.4	7.0
Health Insurance									
Medicaid/CHIP	8.4%*	100.0%	0.4%*	31.0%*	–	100.0%	100.0%	100.0%	100.0%
Medicare	3.4*	12.4	1.0*	100.0*	–	12.4	100.0*	–	–
Private	67.5*	3.1	100.0*	20.9*	–	3.1	1.8	3.8	3.2

See Table 4C for sources and notes.

MACStats

SECTION 2

MACStats

TABLE 4B. Health Characteristics of Non-institutionalized Individuals Age 19-64 by Source of Health Insurance, 2007–2009

	All Non-aged Adults	Selected Sources of Insurance[1]				Medicaid/CHIP non-aged adults	Medicaid/CHIP[2]		
		Medicaid/CHIP[2]	Private[3]	Medicare	Uninsured[4]		Medicare (duals)	Non-dual SSI	Neither SSI nor Medicare
Disability and work status									
Receives SSI	2.3%*	**21.0%**	0.3%*	21.4%	0.4%*	**21.0%**	40.8%*	100.0%*	0.0
Receives SSDI	3.0%*	**13.9**	1.2*	60.3*	0.5*	**13.9**	62.1*	14.5	5.5*
Working	73.7%*	**36.0**	82.8*	12.2*	66.2*	**36.0**	9.5*	9.7*	46.6*
Current health status (categories sum to 100%)									
Excellent or very good	64.3%*	**37.7%**	71.2%*	11.8%*	57.4%*	**37.7%**	9.0%*	17.3%*	47.2%*
Good	24.7*	**30.0**	22.3*	26.9*	30.1	**30.0**	28.2	24.8*	31.6
Fair or poor	11.0*	**32.2**	6.4*	61.3*	12.5*	**32.2**	62.9*	57.9*	21.3*
Health compared to 12 months ago (categories sum to 100%)									
Better	19.3%	**20.1%**	19.6%	16.7%*	18.2%*	**20.1%**	17.9%	20.3%	20.4%
Worse	8.0*	**17.2**	5.9*	25.4*	9.2*	**17.2**	29.8*	21.8*	14.0*
Same	72.8*	**62.8**	74.4*	57.9*	72.6*	**62.8**	52.3*	57.9*	65.6
Activities of daily living (ADLs)									
Help with any personal care needs[5]	1.2%*	**6.7%**	0.5%*	13.3%*	0.5%*	**6.7%**	19.0%*	13.7%*	2.9%*
Help with bathing/showering	0.7*	**4.5**	0.3*	8.3*	0.2*	**4.5**	12.7*	9.7*	1.9*
Help with dressing	0.7*	**3.9**	0.3*	7.9*	0.2*	**3.9**	12.0*	8.0*	1.6*
Help with eating	0.2*	**1.5**	0.1*	2.3	0.1*	**1.5**	3.9*	3.8*	0.6*
Help with transferring (in/out of bed or chairs)	0.6*	**3.5**	0.3*	7.3*	0.2*	**3.5**	9.5*	6.7*	1.7*
Help with toileting	0.4*	**2.6**	0.1*	5.2*	0.1*	**2.6**	8.2*	5.2*	1.0*
Help getting around in home	0.5*	**2.7**	0.2*	5.3*	0.1*	**2.7**	7.1*	4.1	1.6*
Number of above ADLs reported (categories sum to 100%)									
0	99.0%*	**94.3%**	99.6%*	88.6%*	99.7%*	**94.3%**	83.6%*	88.1%*	97.5%*
1	0.2%*	**0.8**	0.1*	1.9*	0.1*	**0.8**	2.2*	2.4*	0.3*
2	0.2*	**1.5**	0.1*	2.7*	0.1*	**1.5**	3.9*	3.0	0.7*
3	0.2*	**0.9**	0.1*	2.2*	0.0*	**0.9**	3.1*	1.5	0.4*
4+	0.4*	**2.4**	0.2*	4.6*	0.1*	**2.4**	7.1*	4.9*	1.1*

Updated on July 25, 2011. Table 4B reflects corrections to typographical errors found after the Report's publication.

TABLE 4B, Continued

	All Non-aged Adults	Selected Sources of Insurance[1]				Medicaid/CHIP non-aged adults	Medicaid/CHIP[2]		
		Medicaid/ CHIP[2]	Private[3]	Medicare	Uninsured[4]		Medicare (duals)	Non-dual SSI	Neither SSI nor Medicare
Specific health conditions									
Currently pregnant	1.3%*	4.8%	1.1%*	†	0.7%*	4.8%	†	0.9%*	6.5%*
Functional limitation[6]	27.2*	48.5	23.7*	82.8%*	24.5*	48.5	83.2%*	75.2*	36.7*
Difficulty walking without equipment	3.2*	12.6	1.7*	33.5*	1.8*	12.6	36.0*	23.9*	6.1*
Health condition that requires special equipment (e.g., cane, wheelchair)	3.9*	13.3	2.5*	33.0*	2.0*	13.3	36.1*	25.2*	6.7*
Lost all natural teeth	4.6*	9.6	3.4*	18.4*	4.9*	9.6	20.3*	16.8*	6.1*
Depressed/anxious feelings[7]	11.6*	28.0	7.7*	34.8*	15.7*	28.0	43.3*	39.1*	23.1*
Ever told had hypertension	22.4*	32.2	21.8*	55.0*	17.1*	32.2	55.8*	46.7*	24.8*
Ever told had coronary heart disease	2.3*	4.2	2.0*	13.4*	1.3*	4.2	10.2*	7.6*	2.5*
Ever told had heart attack	1.8*	3.9	1.4*	10.5*	1.2*	3.9	8.9*	7.6*	2.2*
Ever told had stroke	1.4*	4.4	0.9*	11.5*	1.0*	4.4	10.7*	8.1*	2.4*
Ever told had cancer	4.9*	6.1	5.1*	11.5*	2.9*	6.1	11.4*	9.6*	4.5*
Ever told had diabetes	6.4*	12.7	5.7*	25.9*	4.8*	12.7	30.2*	19.4*	8.1*
Ever told had arthritis	17.0*	24.8	17.0*	51.2*	10.8*	24.8	50.1*	38.9*	17.3*
Ever told had asthma	12.4*	19.7	11.8*	21.0	11.2*	19.7	26.4*	27.0*	16.9*
Past 12 months, told had chronic bronchitis	3.7*	8.1	3.0*	12.5*	3.7*	8.1	13.6*	13.9*	5.9*
Past 12 months, told had liver condition	1.4*	3.5	1.0*	6.0*	1.3*	3.5	7.8*	6.1*	2.1*
Past 12 months, told had weak/failing kidneys	1.2*	4.2	0.7*	8.1*	1.2*	4.2	9.8*	6.8*	2.7*

See Table 4C for sources and notes.

Updated on July 25, 2011. Table 4B reflects corrections to typographical errors found after the Report's publication.

MACStats

SECTION 2

MACStats

TABLE 4C.   Use of Care by Non-institutionalized Individuals Age 19-64 by Source of Health Insurance, 2007–2009

	All Non-aged Adults	Selected Sources of Insurance[1]				Medicaid/CHIP non-aged adults	Medicaid/CHIP[2]		
		Medicaid/CHIP[2]	Private[3]	Medicare	Uninsured[4]		Medicare (duals)	Non-dual SSI	Neither SSI nor Medicare
Received at-home care in past 12 months	1.2%*	5.2%	0.9%*	9.1%*	0.4%*	5.2%	14.6%*	9.3%*	2.5%*
Number of times saw a doctor or other health professional in past 12 months (categories sum to 100%)									
None	21.6%*	13.9%	15.5%*	6.2%*	46.9%*	13.9%	3.2%*	8.9%*	16.9%*
1	18.2%*	11.4	19.2%	6.6*	18.7*	11.4	3.4*	8.3*	13.5*
2-3	26.6%*	20.7	30.3*	15.6*	17.3*	20.7	15.1*	16.0*	22.6
4+	33.7*	54.0	35.1*	71.5*	17.1*	54.0	78.3*	66.8*	47.0*
Number of emergency room visits in past 12 months (categories sum to 100%)									
None	80.1%*	59.8%	83.4%*	59.0%	79.4%*	59.8%	54.0%	53.1%*	62.3%
1	12.6%*	18.5	11.7*	19.3	12.5*	18.5	18.8	20.0	18.1
2-3	5.3*	13.0	3.9*	13.2	6.0*	13.0	15.6	15.2	12.1
4+	2.0*	8.7	1.0*	8.4	2.1*	8.7	11.5	11.7*	7.5

Notes: Health insurance coverage is defined at the time of the survey. Totals of health insurance coverage may sum to more than 100% because individuals may have multiple sources of coverage. Responses to recent care questions are based on the previous 12 months, during which time the individual may have had different coverage than that shown in the table. Not separately shown are the estimates of individuals covered by any type of military health plan (VA, TRICARE, and CHAMP-VA) or other government programs. In order to focus on a consistent sample across the measures included in this table, the tabulations reported here are based on the NHIS sample adult weights. Somewhat different estimates might be obtained using the broader person file weights for the subset of variables that are available for all persons in the household. This analysis provides conservative estimates of statistical significance; it does not take into account subgroups' non-independence by incorporating the covariance.

† Estimates with a relative standard error of greater than 50% are indicated with a dagger and are not shown.

* Difference from Medicaid/CHIP is statistically significant at the 95 percent confidence level

– Quantity zero; amounts shown as 0.0 round to less than 0.1 in this table.

1 Not separately shown are the estimates of individuals covered by any type of military health plan (VA, TRICARE, and CHAMP-VA) or other government programs.

2 Medicaid/CHIP health insurance coverage also includes persons covered by other state-sponsored health plans. Federal surveys such as NHIS do not publish separate results for Medicaid and CHIP enrollment. CHIP enrollment of adults is small, totaling less than 350,000 ever enrolled during FY 2010 (March 2011 MACStats).

3 Private health insurance coverage excludes plans that paid for only one type of service, such as accidents or dental care.

4 A person was defined as uninsured if he/she did not have any private health insurance, Medicare, Medicaid, CHIP, state-sponsored or other government-sponsored health plans, or military plan. A person was also defined as uninsured if he/she had only Indian Health Service (IHS) coverage or had only a private plan that paid for one type of service, such as accidents or dental care.

5 Only adults who report needing assistance with personal care needs are asked about each of the following specific personal care needs. Each specific personal care need is reported as the overall population incidence (rather than the incidence among those needing help with any personal care needs).

6 Individuals with a functional limitation are those who reported any degree of difficulty—ranging from "only a little difficult" to "can't do at all"—doing any of a dozen activities (e.g., walking a quarter of a mile, stooping or kneeling) by themselves and without special equipment.

7 Reports feeling sad, hopeless, worthless, nervous, restless, or that everything was an effort all or most of the time.

Source: Urban Institute analysis of the National Health Interview Survey (NHIS) for MACPAC; the estimates for 2007–2009 are based on household interviews of a sample of the civilian non-institutionalized population.

The NHIS analysis file for sample adults had been previously constructed with funding under the Robert Wood Johnson Foundation's State Health Access Reform Evaluation (SHARE) initiative as part of another project. We appreciate Sharon Long's willingness to share that file with MACPAC.

TABLE 5A. Health Insurance and Demographic Characteristics of Non-institutionalized Individuals Age 65 and Older by Source of Health Insurance, 2007–2009

| | All Aged Adults | Selected Sources of Insurance[1] | | | All Medicaid aged adults | Medicaid[2] | |
		Medicaid[2]	Private[3]	Medicare		Functional limitation[4]	No functional limitation
Health Insurance Coverage		**7.3%**	57.4%	95.2%	**100.0%**	76.8%	23.2%
Age (categories sum to 100%)							
65-74	53.7%	**53.4%**	53.5%	52.5%	**53.4%**	51.2%	61.0%
75-84	34.7	**36.0**	34.7	35.6	**36.0**	36.3	35.3
85+	11.6	**10.6**	11.8	11.9	**10.6**	12.6	3.7*
Gender (categories sum to 100%)							
Male	43.1%*	**33.7%**	43.4%*	42.6%*	**33.7%**	29.7%	47.3%*
Female	56.9*	**66.3**	56.6*	57.4*	**66.3**	70.3	52.7*
Race (categories sum to 100%)							
Hispanic	6.9%*	**23.1%**	3.0%*	6.5%*	**23.1%**	22.3%	25.7%
White, non-Hispanic	80.0*	**47.2**	87.8*	80.9*	**47.2**	49.3	40.5
Black, non-Hispanic	8.4*	**18.3**	5.5*	8.2*	**18.3**	19.6	13.4*
Other and multiple races, non-Hispanic	4.7*	**11.4**	3.6*	4.4*	**11.4**	8.7	20.4*
Health insurance							
Medicaid/CHIP	7.3%*	**100.0%**	0.7%*	7.0%*	**100.0%**	100.0%	100.0%
Medicare	95.2*	**91.0**	94.6*	100.0*	**91.0**	91.7	89.2
Private	57.4*	**5.3**	100.0*	57.0*	**5.3**	4.7	6.8

See Table 5C for sources and notes.

Updated on July 25, 2011. Table 5A reflects corrections to typographical errors found after the Report's publication.

MACStats

SECTION 2

MACStats

SECTION 2

TABLE 5B. Health Characteristics of Non-institutionalized Individuals Age 65 and Older by Source of Health Insurance, 2007–2009

	All Aged Adults	Selected Sources of Insurance[1]			All Medicaid aged adults	Medicaid[2]	
		Medicaid[2]	Private[3]	Medicare		Functional limitation[4]	No functional limitation
Disability and work status							
Receives SSI	3.8%*	37.4%	0.5%*	3.8%*	37.4%	37.8%	34.8%
Working	15.0*	4.2	17.8*	13.7*	4.2	2.5	9.5*
Current health status (categories sum to 100%)							
Excellent or very good	40.7%*	16.1%	44.8%*	40.4%*	16.1%	10.8%*	33.8%*
Good	34.3	32.4	35.3	34.4	32.4	29.5	42.4*
Fair or poor	25.1*	51.5	19.9*	25.2*	51.5	59.7*	23.7*
Health compared to 12 months ago (categories sum to 100%)							
Better	13.4%	13.4%	13.3%	13.3%	13.4%	13.2%	13.9%
Worse	12.7*	22.1	11.4*	12.8*	22.1	26.3*	7.9*
Same	73.8*	64.6	75.3*	73.9*	64.6	60.4	78.2*
Activities of daily living (ADLs)							
Help with any personal care needs[5]	6.4%*	18.7%	4.6%*	6.6%*	18.7%	23.0%	4.3%*
Help with bathing/showering	4.7*	15.3	3.3*	4.8*	15.3	18.9	3.0*
Help with dressing	3.8*	11.5	2.7*	3.9*	11.5	14.3	2.3*
Help with eating	1.5*	5.0	1.0*	1.5*	5.0	6.1	1.4*
Help with transferring (in/out of bed or chairs)	2.9*	9.3	1.9*	3.0*	9.3	11.3	2.1*
Help with toileting	2.2*	7.2	1.5*	2.3*	7.2	8.8	1.4*
Help getting around in home	2.6*	8.2	1.8*	2.7*	8.2	10.1	1.4*
Number of above ADLs reported (categories sum to 100%)							
0	94.1%*	82.5%	95.9%*	94.0%*	82.5%	78.2%	97.0%
1	1.6*	3.5	1.4*	1.7*	3.5	4.4	†
2	1.3*	4.6	0.8*	1.3*	4.6	6.0	†
3	0.7*	2.3	0.5*	0.8*	2.3	2.8	†
4+	2.2*	7.0	1.5*	2.2*	7.0	8.6	1.4*

Updated on July 25, 2011. Table 5B reflects corrections to typographical errors found after the Report's publication.

TABLE 5B, Continued

	All Aged Adults	Selected Sources of Insurance[1]			Medicaid[2]		
		Medicaid[2]	Private[3]	Medicare	All Medicaid aged adults	Functional limitation[4]	No functional limitation[4]
Specific health conditions							
Functional limitation[4]	62.9%*	76.8%	61.9%*	63.5%*	76.8%	100.0%*	0.0%*
Difficulty walking without equipment	18.6*	35.2	16.3*	18.9*	35.2	43.3*	6.6*
Health condition that requires special equipment (e.g., cane, wheelchair)	19.8*	34.8	17.5*	20.2*	34.8	43.3*	7.0*
Lost all natural teeth	25.2*	42.9	21.5*	25.3*	42.9	45.5	34.5*
Depressed/anxious feelings[6]	9.3*	22.3	7.3*	9.4*	22.3	26.0	10.5*
Ever told had hypertension	61.4*	70.9	60.9*	62.0*	70.9	74.9	57.0*
Ever told had coronary heart disease	15.0*	19.1	15.2*	15.2*	19.1	21.3	12.1*
Ever told had heart attack	11.8*	16.1	11.2*	11.9*	16.1	17.5	11.8
Ever told had stroke	8.9*	13.1	8.4*	9.1*	13.1	16.2*	3.0*
Ever told had cancer	23.2*	18.2	26.1*	23.5*	18.2	20.4	10.0*
Ever told had diabetes	18.9*	29.2	16.9*	19.1*	29.2	33.2	16.0*
Ever told had arthritis	50.0*	57.5	50.3*	50.6*	57.5	66.4*	27.8*
Ever told had asthma	10.7*	14.3	10.5*	10.7*	14.3	15.7	9.7
Past 12 months, told had chronic bronchitis	5.7*	9.6	5.1*	5.8*	9.6	11.1	4.7*
Past 12 months, told had liver condition	1.4*	3.1	1.3*	1.5*	3.1	3.3	†
Past 12 months, told had weak/failing kidneys	4.3*	8.2	3.8*	4.4*	8.2	9.2	4.3*

See Table 5C for sources and notes.

Updated on July 25, 2011. Table 5B reflects corrections to typographical errors found after the Report's publication

MACStats

MACStats

TABLE 5C. Use of Care by Non-institutionalized Individuals Age 65 and Older by Source of Health Insurance, 2007–2009

	All Aged Adults	Selected Sources of Insurance[1]			Medicaid[2]		
		Medicaid[2]	Private[3]	Medicare	All Medicaid aged adults	Functional limitation[4]	No functional limitation
Received at-home care in past 12 months	7.3%*	19.0%	6.4%*	7.5%*	19.0%	23.0%	6.0%*
Number of times saw a doctor or other health professional in past 12 months (categories sum to 100%)							
None	6.4%	6.2%	5.0%	6.0%	6.2%	3.8%*	14.1%*
1	9.8	8.0	9.9	9.4	8.0	6.4	13.3*
2-3	24.7*	16.5	26.0*	24.8*	16.5	14.1	24.5*
4+	59.1*	69.2	59.0*	59.7*	69.2	75.6*	48.1*
Number of emergency room visits in past 12 months (categories sum to 100%)							
None	76.2%*	66.3%	77.8%*	75.9%*	66.3%	62.6%	78.5%*
1	15.0	16.4	14.9	15.1	16.4	17.0	14.5
2-3	6.6*	12.2	5.5*	6.8*	12.2	14.4	5.1*
4+	2.2*	5.1	1.9*	2.3*	5.1	6.0	2.0*

Notes: Health insurance coverage is defined at the time of the survey. Totals of health insurance coverage may sum to more than 100% because individuals may have multiple sources of coverage. Responses to recent care questions are based on the previous 12 months, during which time the individual may have had different coverage than that shown in the table. Not separately shown are the estimates of individuals covered by any type of military health plan (VA, TRICARE, and CHAMP-VA) or other government programs. In order to focus on a consistent sample across the measures included in this table, the tabulations reported here are based on the NHIS sample adult weights. Somewhat different estimates might be obtained using the broader person file weights for the subset of variables that are available for all persons in the household. This analysis provides conservative estimates of statistical significance; it does not take into account subgroups' non-independence by incorporating the covariance.

† Estimates with a relative standard error of greater than 50% are indicated with a dagger and are not shown.

* Difference from Medicaid/CHIP is statistically significant at the 95 percent confidence level

– Quantity zero; amounts shown as 0.0 round to less than 0.1 in this table.

1 Not separately shown are the estimates of individuals covered by any type of military health plan (VA, TRICARE, and CHAMP-VA) or other government programs. Also not shown are estimates of the aged uninsured (0.6%). The sample size is not sufficient to support published estimates of their characteristics. A person was defined as uninsured if he/she did not have any private health insurance, Medicare, Medicaid, CHIP, state-sponsored or other government-sponsored health plans, or military plan. A person was also defined as uninsured if he/she had only Indian Health Service (IHS) coverage or had only a private plan that paid for one type of service, such as accidents or dental care.

2 Medicaid health insurance coverage also includes persons covered by other public programs, excluding Medicare (e.g., other state-sponsored health plans). Even though survey estimates are generally not published separately for Medicaid and CHIP, CHIP is not shown in the labels of this portion of the NHIS estimates because its occurrence among those aged 65 and older would be rare. Enrollment in CHIP-financed coverage is prohibited for those with other coverage, such as Medicare, and 95% of those 65 and older have Medicare.

3 Private health insurance coverage excludes plans that paid for only one type of service, such as accidents or dental care.

4 Individuals with a functional limitation are those who reported any degree of difficulty—ranging from "only a little difficult" to "can't do at all"—doing any of a dozen activities (e.g., walking a quarter of a mile, stooping or kneeling) by themselves and without special equipment.

5 Only adults who report needing assistance with personal care needs are asked about each of the following specific personal care needs. Each specific personal care need is reported as the overall population incidence (rather than the incidence among those needing help with any personal care needs).

6 Reports feeling sad, hopeless, worthless, nervous, restless, or that everything was an effort all or most of the time.

Source: Urban Institute analysis of the National Health Interview Survey (NHIS); the estimates for 2007-2009 are based on household interviews of a sample of the civilian non-institutionalized population

Medicaid Enrollment and Spending (Tables 6–8 and Figures 3–7)

Tables 6 to 8 and Figures 3 to 7 show Medicaid enrollment and spending, with various breakouts by state, eligibility group, dual eligible status, and type of service. They are based on Medicaid Statistical Information System (MSIS) data for FY 2008 (the most recent available for all states) that have been adjusted to match benefit spending totals reported by states in CMS-64, as discussed in Section 4 of MACStats.

Medicaid benefit spending varies widely across populations:

- Non-disabled adults and children represent the majority of Medicaid enrollees nationally and within each state (Table 6), but disabled and aged enrollees account for the largest share of the program's spending on benefits (Table 7).

- Disabled and aged enrollees have per person Medicaid benefit spending that is 3 to 5 times larger than that of other enrollees (Figure 4 and Table 8).

- Individuals age 65 and older account for about 60 percent of dual eligible enrollment and dual eligible Medicaid benefit spending; younger dual eligibles account for the remaining 40 percent (Tables 6 and 7).

- Spending by type of service also varies among populations: a higher share of spending for disabled and aged enrollees goes to cover long-term services and supports, while a substantial portion of spending for non-disabled children and adults goes to managed care payments (Figures 3 and 4).

- The users of long-term services and supports (LTSS)—primarily disabled and aged enrollees—account for a small share of Medicaid enrollees, but a large share of Medicaid spending on both LTSS and acute care (Figures 4 through 7).

Medicaid benefit spending per enrollee also varies substantially across states (Table 8). Reasons for this variation may include the breadth of benefits that states choose to cover; the portion of enrollees receiving a full benefit package or a more limited version; enrollee case mix (based on health status and other characteristics); the underlying cost of delivering health care services in a geographic area; and state policies regarding provider payments, care management, and other issues.

Information reported by states in MSIS indicates that the portion of enrollees receiving limited benefits ranged from less than 2 percent in five states to more than 20 percent in another three in FY 2008 (Table 8). These percentages vary by enrollee population; for example, in many states with family planning waivers, a substantial portion of non-disabled adult enrollees received limited benefits.[32]

Even when comparisons are limited to similar populations, Medicaid spending per enrollee still varies substantially across states. For example, one analysis of disabled enrollees with similar income levels (i.e., low enough to qualify for cash assistance under the SSI program) receiving full Medicaid-only fee-for-service benefits (i.e., excluding enrollees with limited benefits, those with Medicare coverage, and those in managed care) found that Medicaid spending per enrollee on acute care in the highest spending state was more than double the

---

[32] In FY 2008, the following states had implemented waivers providing Medicaid coverage limited to family planning: AL, AZ, AR, CA, DE, FL, IA, IL, LA, MD, MI, MN, MO, MS, NY, NC, NM, OK, OR, PA, RI, SC, TX, VA, WA, and WI. See CMS, *Section 1115 Demonstrations, State Profiles: Approvals Through January 31, 2009* (Baltimore, MD: CMS).

SECTION 2

amount in the lowest spending state.[33] It also found that most of the cross-state variation in Medicaid spending per enrollee was a result of differences in the quantity of services provided rather than the unit price of services, that LTSS Medicaid spending per enrollee varied more than acute care, and that variation in Medicaid spending per enrollee exceeded that of Medicare.

MACStats

---

[33] See Robert Wood Johnson Foundation, *Geographic variation and health care cost growth: Research to inform a complex diagnosis* (Washington, DC: AcademyHealth, October 2009). http://www.academyhealth.org/files/HCFO/HCFOPolicyBriefOCT09.pdf; and R. Kronick and T. Gilmer, Inter- and intrastate variation in Medicaid expenditures, presentation at the AcademyHealth Annual Research Meeting, June 28, 2009, http://www.academyhealth. org/files/2009/sunday/KronickR.pdf.

MAC Stats

MACStats

TABLE 6. Medicaid Enrollment by State, Eligibility Group, and Dual Eligible Status, FY 2008 (thousands)

| State | Total | Percentage of Enrollees in Eligibility Group[1] | | | | Dual Eligible Status[2] | | | | | |
| | | Children | Adults | Disabled | Aged | All duals | | Duals with full benefits | | Duals with limited benefits | |
						Total	Percentage age 65+[3]	Total	Percentage age 65+[3]	Total	Percentage age 65+[3]
Total	**58,800**	**48.2%**	**26.1%**	**16.5%**	**9.1%**	**9,155**	**60.9%**	**7,134**	**60.9%**	**2,021**	**61.0%**
Alabama	909	48.2	16.2	24.3	11.3	208	58.9	100	54.2	108	63.3
Alaska	113	56.5	23.0	14.0	6.4	13	54.7	13	54.2	0	73.3
Arizona	1,539	45.7	39.6	9.2	5.4	148	58.8	115	55.1	33	71.6
Arkansas	685	52.4	18.2	19.2	10.2	118	56.1	69	61.2	50	49.1
California	10,590	39.0	42.6	10.9	7.5	1,201	70.8	1,175	70.6	27	77.6
Colorado	572	58.3	17.4	14.8	9.5	83	60.3	68	60.0	15	61.7
Connecticut	553	52.1	23.7	12.2	12.0	103	61.4	78	59.5	25	67.4
Delaware	192	42.5	38.6	12.0	6.9	24	55.5	11	54.4	13	56.5
District of Columbia	163	45.2	25.5	23.4	6.0	22	60.6	19	60.5	3	61.5
Florida	3,021	50.5	18.8	18.5	12.2	601	66.0	349	69.0	253	61.8
Georgia	1,683	57.6	17.3	17.0	8.2	264	60.5	146	61.0	118	59.9
Hawaii	219	41.9	35.9	11.8	10.4	33	69.3	30	70.0	3	62.4
Idaho	205	60.8	13.1	18.2	8.0	31	50.4	22	50.2	9	51.0
Illinois	2,390	56.2	22.3	14.5	7.1	313	58.0	275	57.1	39	64.1
Indiana	1,049	55.8	21.1	15.0	8.1	156	50.9	101	54.9	55	43.8
Iowa	475	46.5	29.0	15.5	8.9	81	52.3	68	49.9	13	65.1
Kansas	355	56.0	14.8	19.1	10.1	63	52.9	47	54.4	16	48.7
Kentucky	841	46.0	16.3	29.1	8.6	178	53.0	110	53.9	68	51.6
Louisiana	1,055	52.7	17.6	19.3	10.4	180	60.1	107	58.0	73	63.1
Maine	344	34.9	31.3	17.3	16.5	92	61.3	53	48.2	39	79.3
Maryland	753	49.0	24.2	18.9	7.9	110	59.2	74	60.0	35	57.4
Massachusetts	1,489	29.0	26.5	33.7	10.8	255	53.9	248	52.7	7	95.6
Michigan	1,919	55.4	21.2	16.3	7.1	264	50.5	234	50.1	30	54.0
Minnesota	808	48.4	25.5	14.5	11.6	132	56.0	120	54.8	12	67.4
Mississippi	737	49.4	16.9	23.3	10.4	151	58.5	81	60.9	69	55.8
Missouri	988	53.1	18.7	18.7	9.3	172	51.3	156	51.1	16	54.0
Montana	110	54.5	18.8	18.1	8.7	18	56.7	16	54.4	3	71.0
Nebraska	227	54.7	19.2	15.6	10.4	42	54.3	38	53.5	4	61.4
Nevada	260	55.6	19.8	15.4	9.2	40	60.6	22	65.6	18	54.6
New Hampshire	148	60.0	13.8	16.1	10.1	29	49.1	21	49.5	8	47.9
New Jersey	953	53.4	13.9	20.8	11.9	204	66.8	175	66.2	28	70.4

TABLE 6, Continued

State	Percentage of Enrollees in Eligibility Group[1]					Dual Eligible Status[2]					
						All duals		Duals with full benefits		Duals with limited benefits	
	Total	Children	Adults	Disabled	Aged	Total	Percentage age 65+[3]	Total	Percentage age 65+[3]	Total	Percentage age 65+[3]
New Mexico	506	61.0%	20.2%	13.6%	5.3%	56	61.5%	40	61.4%	16	61.7%
New York	4,937	39.3	36.4	15.1	9.2	737	68.9	659	67.7	79	78.8
North Carolina	1,684	51.8	19.8	17.5	10.8	310	57.6	250	57.2	60	59.5
North Dakota	71	50.3	21.4	15.4	12.9	15	59.4	11	59.3	4	59.7
Ohio	1,947	46.5	25.2	18.6	9.6	304	52.1	205	54.3	98	47.4
Oklahoma	723	56.5	19.4	15.1	9.0	114	56.9	95	56.8	19	57.7
Oregon	520	50.7	23.0	16.5	9.8	90	56.6	62	58.1	28	53.1
Pennsylvania	2,199	45.3	19.6	24.4	10.7	392	56.5	333	55.3	59	62.9
Rhode Island	186	46.0	18.9	23.7	11.4	39	59.2	34	57.3	6	70.5
South Carolina	840	49.3	23.6	17.9	9.1	151	55.7	132	55.2	19	59.1
South Dakota	120	58.4	17.0	16.1	8.5	21	60.5	14	61.7	7	58.0
Tennessee	1,479	48.7	20.5	24.1	6.6	285	51.4	216	44.6	68	73.0
Texas	4,278	62.7	14.0	13.3	10.1	626	67.6	408	68.6	219	65.7
Utah	295	54.5	27.7	13.0	4.8	31	47.3	28	46.5	3	55.3
Vermont	168	38.8	36.2	14.1	10.9	32	60.7	25	55.1	7	79.7
Virginia	866	53.3	16.2	19.1	11.4	171	58.0	119	60.2	52	52.8
Washington	1,180	54.7	22.2	15.6	7.6	150	54.2	114	56.5	36	47.0
West Virginia	402	47.5	14.7	28.5	9.4	80	51.2	50	51.6	30	50.5
Wisconsin	974	40.9	29.4	15.6	14.0	210	68.4	194	68.5	16	67.6
Wyoming	78	65.1	14.7	13.1	7.1	10	53.9	7	52.5	3	56.7

Notes: Numbers reflect individuals ever enrolled during the year, even if for a single month. Excludes Medicaid-expansion CHIP enrollees and the territories. Estimates based on MSIS APS data may differ slightly from those derived from MSIS state summary data used in MACPAC, *Report to the Congress: March 2011.*

Although more recent state-level information is not available, the estimated number ever enrolled in Medicaid (excluding Medicaid-expansion CHIP) nationally is 62.9 million for FY 2009; 67.7 million for FY 2010; 70.4 million for FY 2011; and 71.7 million for FY 2012. These FY 2009–FY 2012 figures include about one million enrollees in the territories. (Source: Office of the Actuary (OACT), Centers for Medicare & Medicaid Services. *2010 Actuarial Report on the Financial Outlook for Medicaid,* 2010; MACPAC communication with OACT, February 2011.)

1 Children and non-aged adults who qualify for Medicaid on the basis of a disability are included in the disabled category.

2 Dual eligibles with limited benefits receive Medicaid assistance with Medicare premiums and cost sharing only.

3 Some states continue to categorize individuals as disabled after they turn 65; as a result, the number of duals age 65+ may exceed the number who are categorized as aged.

Source: MACPAC analysis of Medicaid Statistical Information System (MSIS) annual person summary (APS) data from CMS as of May 2011

Updated on July 25, 2011; Table 6 reflects the addition of a clarifying footnote after the Report's publication.

SECTION 2

MACStats

TABLE 7. Medicaid Benefit Spending by State, Eligibility Group, and Dual Eligible Status, FY 2008 (millions)

| State | Percentage of Benefit Spending Attributable to Eligibility Group[1] | | | | | Dual Eligible Status[2] | | | | | |
| | | | | | | All duals | | Duals with full benefits | | Duals with limited benefits | |
	Total	Children	Adults	Disabled	Aged	Total	Percentage attributable to age 65+[3]	Total	Percentage attributable to age 65+[3]	Total	Percentage attributable to age 65+[3]
Total	**$338,552**	**20.1%**	**14.6%**	**44.5%**	**20.8%**	**$117,796**	**62.1%**	**$113,725**	**62.4%**	**$4,071**	**54.4%**
Alabama	4,078	27.2	9.9	41.2	21.6	1,586	70.1	1,387	71.4	199	60.9
Alaska	890	26.9	14.2	39.3	19.6	275	60.0	275	60.0	1	55.8
Arizona	7,506	25.7	33.2	30.8	10.2	1,333	56.7	1,286	56.3	48	65.6
Arkansas	3,287	24.4	5.5	44.1	26.0	1,363	59.6	1,183	62.9	180	38.0
California	39,042	16.9	17.6	45.1	20.4	13,196	67.6	13,129	67.6	67	71.5
Colorado	3,169	22.9	11.9	41.4	23.8	1,122	62.8	1,102	62.9	19	57.2
Connecticut	4,544	18.8	9.6	38.8	32.9	2,283	62.3	2,235	62.6	48	51.5
Delaware	1,102	20.0	29.4	33.2	17.3	307	62.1	280	63.3	27	49.4
District of Columbia	1,446	17.7	15.2	53.9	13.2	364	61.6	350	62.5	14	39.8
Florida	14,691	19.5	12.8	45.1	22.7	5,655	63.5	5,104	64.6	552	53.4
Georgia	7,338	26.2	18.3	38.9	16.6	2,016	68.0	1,833	69.4	183	54.4
Hawaii	1,207	15.5	23.2	38.2	23.1	401	69.3	396	69.4	5	58.5
Idaho	1,207	24.7	12.2	46.3	16.9	354	54.3	337	54.7	16	45.6
Illinois	11,602	26.7	13.7	47.7	11.9	3,052	57.3	2,984	57.4	68	52.8
Indiana	6,151	19.7	11.3	48.9	20.0	2,144	55.1	2,033	56.1	111	37.5
Iowa	2,844	18.0	13.5	46.1	22.4	1,220	52.2	1,195	52.2	25	56.2
Kansas	2,274	19.9	8.8	44.2	27.1	883	55.4	857	55.9	27	41.1
Kentucky	4,809	21.1	13.7	48.5	16.8	1,518	64.3	1,398	65.7	121	48.1
Louisiana	6,068	18.8	13.3	50.5	17.4	1,790	57.2	1,646	57.3	143	56.3
Maine	2,253	22.4	14.3	43.7	19.6	794	54.3	735	53.0	58	69.5
Maryland	5,701	19.8	12.2	48.9	19.0	1,800	63.9	1,692	64.7	107	50.9
Massachusetts	10,822	18.2	15.8	42.6	23.4	4,008	59.1	3,997	59.0	11	93.6
Michigan	9,847	21.8	17.1	41.3	19.9	2,996	65.6	2,939	65.9	57	46.1
Minnesota	6,978	19.0	11.2	47.3	22.4	3,004	50.5	2,984	50.5	20	52.7
Mississippi	3,812	20.4	11.2	45.0	23.4	1,448	65.9	1,258	68.2	190	50.9
Missouri	7,090	25.3	11.2	46.4	17.1	2,045	55.7	2,013	55.9	32	42.4
Montana	776	23.8	13.1	39.4	23.7	284	67.8	277	68.1	7	55.0
Nebraska	1,588	24.2	9.6	41.4	24.8	665	55.9	660	56.0	5	47.7
Nevada	1,317	28.0	11.2	43.8	17.0	335	64.2	298	66.4	37	46.4
New Hampshire	1,257	27.5	9.6	36.2	26.7	525	60.7	504	61.0	21	52.2

TABLE 7, Continued

State	Percentage of Benefit Spending Attributable to Eligibility Group[1]					Dual Eligible Status[2]					
						All duals		Duals with full benefits		Duals with limited benefits	
	Total	Children	Adults	Disabled	Aged	Total	Percentage attributable to age 65+[3]	Total	Percentage attributable to age 65+[3]	Total	Percentage attributable to age 65+[3]
New Jersey	9,425	16.3%	8.3%	53.2%	22.1%	4,103	63.2%	4,064	63.2%	39	68.7%
New Mexico	3,045	32.9	14.8	42.5	9.8	712	59.2	683	59.2	30	57.4
New York	47,618	11.3	17.8	47.9	23.0	19,792	61.9	19,611	61.8	181	76.5
North Carolina	10,162	24.3	16.3	42.0	17.5	2,951	59.5	2,858	59.8	93	48.7
North Dakota	534	14.1	10.2	42.2	33.5	299	59.9	293	60.1	6	45.6
Ohio	12,414	13.4	13.5	46.5	26.7	4,573	58.4	4,264	59.5	308	42.7
Oklahoma	3,539	27.3	11.1	41.5	20.1	1,240	56.5	1,217	56.6	22	51.5
Oregon	3,220	20.6	16.3	40.5	22.7	1,148	63.5	1,103	64.2	45	45.5
Pennsylvania	16,300	16.7	10.1	44.1	29.1	6,342	71.6	6,260	71.7	82	58.4
Rhode Island	1,834	19.2	9.6	55.7	15.5	599	53.7	591	53.7	8	54.4
South Carolina	4,437	22.9	15.9	42.8	18.4	1,477	59.3	1,455	59.4	21	54.0
South Dakota	656	24.9	12.5	40.8	21.9	256	64.1	242	64.8	14	51.9
Tennessee	7,176	21.4	16.9	46.9	14.9	2,506	53.6	2,427	53.1	79	70.6
Texas	21,461	34.9	10.3	37.7	17.1	5,385	65.3	4,923	65.2	462	66.5
Utah	1,517	29.4	16.3	43.3	11.0	390	43.9	386	43.9	4	44.3
Vermont	1,080	[4]	[4]	[4]	[4]	[4]		[4]		[4]	
Virginia	5,384	22.5	11.0	45.9	20.6	1,841	58.4	1,735	59.3	106	44.5
Washington	6,293	22.3	14.4	42.1	21.1	1,888	62.8	1,809	63.8	79	41.7
West Virginia	2,278	19.1	9.7	50.1	21.1	792	64.9	741	66.1	51	47.6
Wisconsin	4,989	12.3	14.9	43.5	29.4	2,371	64.5	2,346	64.6	25	55.2
Wyoming	493	25.7	10.4	41.9	22.1	203	52.7	193	52.9	10	49.8

Notes: Includes federal and state funds. Excludes administrative spending, the territories, and Medicaid-expansion CHIP Benefit spending from MSIS data has been adjusted to reflect CMS-64 totals; see Section 4 of MACStats for methodology.

1 Children and non-aged adults who qualify for Medicaid on the basis of a disability are included in the disabled category.

2 Dual eligibles with limited benefits receive Medicare assistance with Medicare premiums and cost-sharing only.

3 Some states continue to categorize individuals as disabled after they turn 65; as a result, the number of duals age 65+ may exceed the number who are categorized as aged.

4 Due to large differences in the way managed care spending is reported by Vermont in CMS-64 and MSIS data, benefit spending based on MACPAC's adjustment methodology is not reported at a level lower than total Medicaid.

Source: MACPAC analysis of Medicaid Statistical Information System (MSIS) annual person summary (APS) data and CMS-64 Financial Management Report (FMR) net expenditure data from CMS as of May 2011.

Updated on July 25, 2011, Table 7 reflects the addition of a clarifying footnote after the Report's publication.

MACStats

SECTION 2

FIGURE 3. Distribution of Medicaid Benefit Spending by Eligibility Group and Service Category, FY 2008

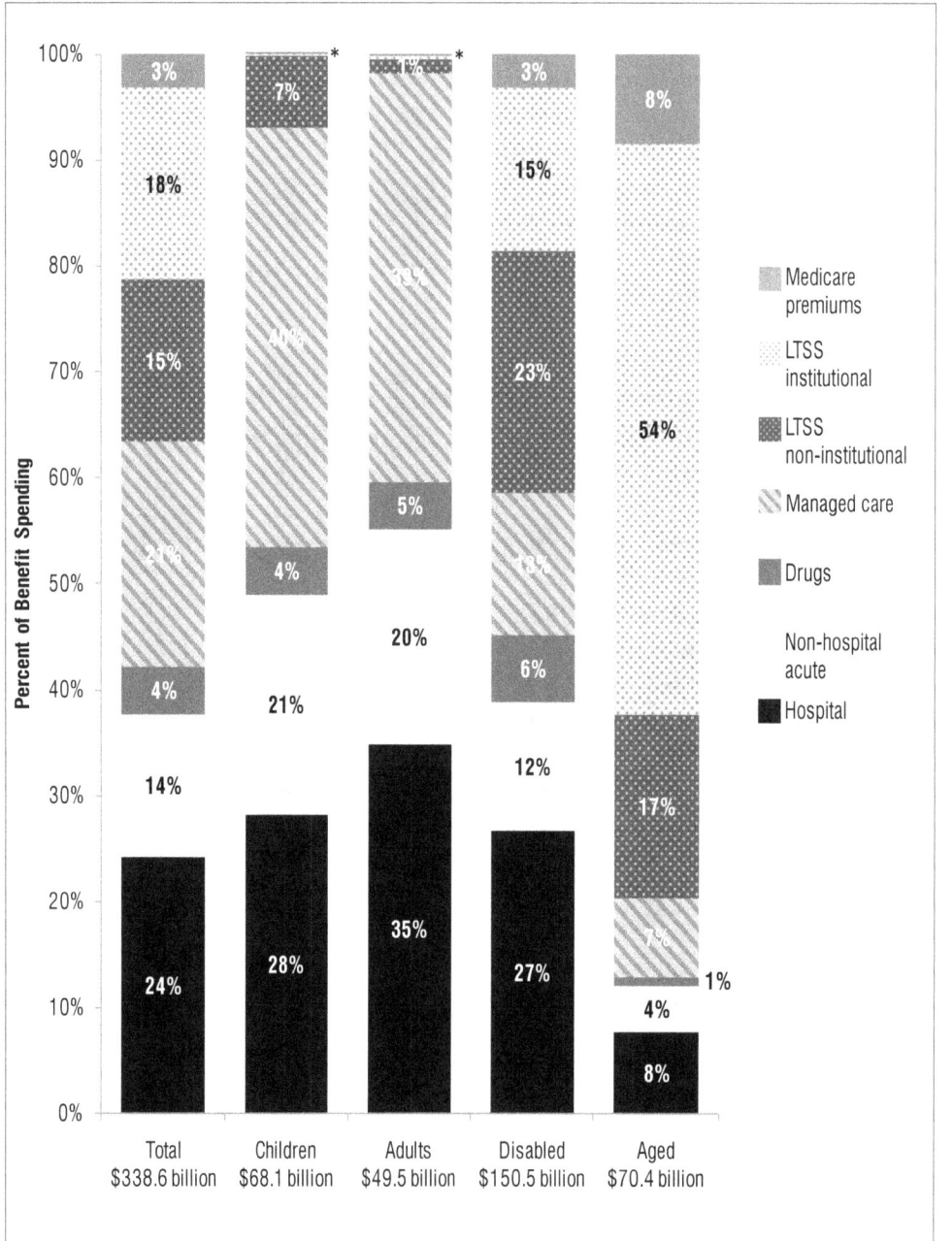

Notes: LTSS = long-term services and supports. Includes federal and state funds. Excludes administrative spending, the territories, and Medicaid-expansion CHIP enrollees. Children and non-aged adults who qualify for Medicaid on the basis of a disability are included in the disabled category. Amounts are fee for service unless otherwise noted. Benefit spending from MSIS data has been adjusted to reflect CMS-64 totals; see Section 4 of MACStats for methodology including a list of services in each category.

*Medicare premiums and LTSS institutional total less than 1%.

Source: MACPAC analysis of Medicaid Statistical Information System (MSIS) annual person summary (APS) data and CMS-64 Financial Management Report (FMR) net expenditure data as of May 2011

MAC Stats

MACStats

TABLE 8. Medicaid Benefit Spending per Full-year Equivalent (FYE) Enrollee by State and Eligibility Group, FY 2008

State	Total — Percentage of FYEs with limited benefits	Total — Benefit Spending per FYE — All enrollees	Total — Benefit Spending per FYE — Excluding those with limited benefits	Children — Percentage of FYEs with limited benefits	Children — Benefit Spending per FYE — All enrollees	Children — Benefit Spending per FYE — Excluding those with limited benefits	Adults — Percentage of FYEs with limited benefits	Adults — Benefit Spending per FYE — All enrollees	Adults — Benefit Spending per FYE — Excluding those with limited benefits	Disabled — Percentage of FYEs with limited benefits	Disabled — Benefit Spending per FYE — All enrollees	Disabled — Benefit Spending per FYE — Excluding those with limited benefits	Aged — Percentage of FYEs with limited benefits	Aged — Benefit Spending per FYE — All enrollees	Aged — Benefit Spending per FYE — Excluding those with limited benefits
Total	11.4%	$7,267	$7,893	1.6%	$3,025	$3,051	29.5%	$4,651	$5,656	8.0%	$17,128	$18,316	23.7%	$15,146	$19,081
Alabama	23.4	5,427	6,315	0.1	3,144	3,143	74.6	3,765	5,901	17.2	8,416	9,688	67.2	9,679	25,500
Alaska	0.3	10,291	10,314	–	4,871	4,871	0.0	7,670	7,666	0.7	24,279	24,421	2.4	26,891	27,511
Arizona	11.0	6,511	6,864	4.4	3,639	3,693	17.9	5,935	6,464	4.4	17,817	17,934	31.7	10,653	14,421
Arkansas	20.2	5,855	6,796	2.1	2,703	2,728	72.1	2,011	5,099	19.0	12,617	14,360	34.8	14,060	19,843
California	29.6	4,829	6,227	8.5	2,076	2,184	66.4	2,193	3,612	0.5	16,384	16,407	5.0	11,328	11,621
Colorado	4.1	7,563	7,650	0.3	3,051	3,012	6.2	6,122	5,592	6.6	18,011	19,056	16.5	16,127	18,971
Connecticut	4.6	9,718	10,081	–	3,497	3,497	0.0	4,129	4,129	11.7	29,197	32,613	25.3	25,909	34,098
Delaware	15.9	7,324	8,248	2.5	3,460	3,518	19.8	6,042	6,850	24.0	17,336	21,954	55.8	16,099	33,881
District of Columbia	2.2	10,439	10,392	0.0	4,072	4,072	0.7	6,514	5,863	3.6	23,332	23,922	18.7	22,720	27,190
Florida	13.7	6,584	7,006	0.0	2,563	2,544	27.9	5,651	5,361	17.3	14,033	16,252	41.3	10,736	16,677
Georgia	8.3	5,811	6,137	0.0	2,662	2,661	0.8	8,101	7,889	16.1	11,203	12,959	51.9	10,147	19,379
Hawaii	1.3	6,685	6,742	0.0	2,356	2,355	0.0	4,827	4,824	3.8	19,623	20,303	7.4	14,102	15,060
Idaho	5.1	7,518	7,813	–	3,058	3,058	0.0	9,663	9,663	11.7	16,508	18,402	29.6	14,421	19,747
Illinois	5.4	5,739	5,938	0.1	2,621	2,620	19.6	4,191	4,646	5.2	17,270	18,069	13.0	9,905	11,156
Indiana	7.5	7,440	7,820	1.2	2,547	2,569	5.6	5,021	4,971	19.2	21,375	25,795	30.2	17,413	23,999
Iowa	10.5	7,640	8,261	1.6	2,969	2,996	26.2	4,032	4,576	5.7	19,174	20,166	20.7	17,659	21,770
Kansas	5.3	8,463	8,803	0.0	3,044	3,041	0.7	6,610	6,409	12.1	16,776	18,793	22.8	20,602	26,209
Kentucky	8.8	7,050	7,525	0.0	3,263	3,259	0.2	7,594	7,555	12.8	10,451	11,663	50.2	13,000	24,238
Louisiana	13.5	6,659	7,305	0.0	2,343	2,342	39.9	5,763	7,674	13.4	16,569	18,718	42.7	10,656	17,183
Maine	11.7	7,682	8,472	0.1	4,993	4,996	0.2	3,716	3,714	12.9	17,876	20,137	53.4	8,733	17,017
Maryland	13.3	9,433	10,102	1.2	3,760	3,744	37.3	5,608	5,325	11.0	21,686	23,853	32.5	21,422	30,216
Massachusetts	1.5	8,665	8,739	0.0	5,434	5,434	0.0	5,372	5,371	0.1	10,774	10,777	12.7	18,041	20,145
Michigan	5.2	6,291	6,550	1.2	2,424	2,447	15.1	5,991	6,871	4.3	14,324	14,823	13.3	16,800	19,026
Minnesota	4.8	11,329	11,826	0.9	4,347	4,373	11.9	5,733	6,333	3.3	31,008	31,967	10.9	23,221	25,896
Mississippi	18.9	6,284	7,062	0.1	2,723	2,722	53.4	4,469	6,353	18.6	11,029	12,767	49.6	12,846	22,822
Missouri	5.8	8,799	9,084	0.1	4,101	4,100	25.8	6,140	6,584	3.8	20,424	21,108	9.3	15,594	16,993
Montana	2.3	9,542	9,679	–	4,161	4,161	0.0	7,940	7,939	3.0	18,317	18,685	17.8	24,465	29,210
Nebraska	1.9	8,878	9,020	–	3,755	3,755	0.0	6,221	6,221	4.1	20,608	21,398	10.2	19,642	21,747
Nevada	8.7	7,071	$7,357	0.3	3,585	3,579	3.0	4,958	4,449	21.2	17,326	20,978	39.0	11,004	16,512

TABLE 8, Continued

State	Total Benefit Spending per FTE			Children Benefit Spending per FTE			Adults Benefit Spending per FTE			Disabled Benefit Spending per FTE			Aged Benefit Spending per FTE		
	Percentage of FTEs with limited benefits[1]	All enrollees	Excluding those with limited benefits[2]	Percentage of FTEs with limited benefits[1]	All enrollees	Excluding those with limited benefits[2]	Percentage of FTEs with limited benefits[1]	All enrollees	Excluding those with limited benefits[2]	Percentage of FTEs with limited benefits[1]	All enrollees	Excluding those with limited benefits[2]	Percentage of FTEs with limited benefits[1]	All enrollees	Excluding those with limited benefits[2]
New Hampshire	5.7%	$10,851	$11,315	–	$4,927	$4,927	0.0	$9,382	$9,383	16.5%	$22,174	$25,969	26.3%	$27,333	$35,862
New Jersey	3.6	11,719	11,947	0.0%	3,577	3,574	1.9%	8,643	7,616	4.4	27,203	28,350	19.2	21,121	25,674
New Mexico	11.1	7,132	7,651	0.0	3,844	3,836	41.3	5,580	7,207	8.8	20,678	22,430	37.8	13,056	19,792
New York	2.9	11,706	11,909	0.8	3,381	3,392	2.7	6,099	6,191	2.0	32,727	33,157	13.4	28,085	31,641
North Carolina	7.5	7,614	7,993	0.1	3,542	3,538	21.7	7,937	9,026	8.2	15,884	17,065	19.7	10,973	13,303
North Dakota	6.6	10,137	10,729	–	2,922	2,922	0.0	5,650	5,649	14.4	23,430	26,970	27.4	23,513	31,879
Ohio	5.4	7,787	8,025	–	2,180	2,180	0.0	4,672	4,672	14.1	18,127	20,454	26.1	21,122	27,435
Oklahoma	7.1	6,412	6,761	0.0	2,985	2,985	30.4	5,164	6,535	6.8	15,199	16,172	16.4	12,701	14,941
Oregon	11.0	8,272	9,017	3.9	3,494	3,592	13.6	6,664	7,104	15.2	16,986	19,652	29.2	16,511	22,671
Pennsylvania	4.2	9,120	9,424	0.2	3,404	3,401	7.1	5,478	5,725	4.0	14,782	15,290	16.3	23,592	27,830
Rhode Island	4.0	11,626	11,952	0.0	4,937	4,932	5.2	6,275	6,262	2.6	25,205	25,715	21.2	15,864	19,578
South Carolina	11.9	6,422	6,913	0.3	3,005	3,006	44.5	4,840	6,230	4.7	13,704	14,289	14.2	11,968	13,744
South Dakota	6.2	6,933	7,230	0.0	2,941	2,941	0.1	6,267	6,254	17.3	15,332	17,962	33.3	16,557	23,764
Tennessee	4.8	5,735	5,950	0.0	2,545	2,543	0.2	5,302	5,284	6.0	10,014	10,562	46.0	12,646	22,345
Texas	6.5	6,702	6,815	0.0	3,768	3,742	2.2	7,232	6,063	13.5	15,656	17,571	33.6	9,393	12,718
Utah	1.5	7,612	7,540	0.1	4,145	4,135	1.4	5,249	4,751	3.7	20,014	20,621	9.2	14,250	15,324
Vermont	4.9	8,051	[3]	–	[3]	[3]	–	[3]	[3]	5.9	[3]	[3]	32.9	[3]	[3]
Virginia	8.0	7,609	7,968	0.0	3,224	3,220	11.4	6,193	6,243	14.6	16,459	18,692	27.3	12,813	16,704
Washington	9.6	6,691	7,130	0.2	2,654	2,651	34.2	5,192	6,880	10.1	16,586	17,961	18.3	17,361	20,562
West Virginia	8.0	7,031	7,467	0.0	2,838	2,838	0.0	6,197	6,192	12.4	11,138	12,415	40.1	14,717	23,335
Wisconsin	9.3	6,346	6,834	1.2	1,960	1,967	25.7	3,473	4,156	3.0	15,431	15,806	8.5	12,290	13,301
Wyoming	5.5	8,478	8,756	0.7	3,341	3,355	3.8	7,535	7,590	13.1	23,267	26,110	33.4	23,583	33,793

Notes: Includes federal and state funds. Excludes administrative spending, the territories, and Medicaid-expansion CHIP. Children and non-aged adults who qualify for Medicaid on the basis of a disability are included in the disabled category. Benefit spending from MSIS data has been adjusted to reflect CMS-64 totals; see Section 4 of MACStats for methodology.

In this table, enrollees with limited benefits are defined as those reported by states in MSIS as receiving coverage of only family planning services; assistance with Medicare premiums and cost sharing; or emergency services. Additional individuals may receive limited benefits for other reasons, but are not broken out here.

– Quantity zero; amounts shown as 0.0 round to less than 0.1 in this table.

1 These percentages are likely to be underestimated because comparisons with other data sources indicate that some states do not identify all of their limited benefit enrollees in MSIS.

2 Calculated by removing limited benefit enrollees and their spending.

3 Due to large differences in the way managed care spending is reported by Vermont in CMS-64 and MSIS data, benefit spending based on MACPAC's adjustment methodology is not reported at a level lower than total Medicaid.

Source: MACPAC analysis of Medicaid Statistical Information System (MSIS) annual person summary (APS) data and CMS-64 Financial Management Report (FMR) net expenditure data from CMS as of May 2011.

MACStats

SECTION 2

MACStats

FIGURE 4. Medicaid Benefit Spending Per Full-year Equivalent (FYE) Enrollee by Eligibility Group and Service Category, FY 2008

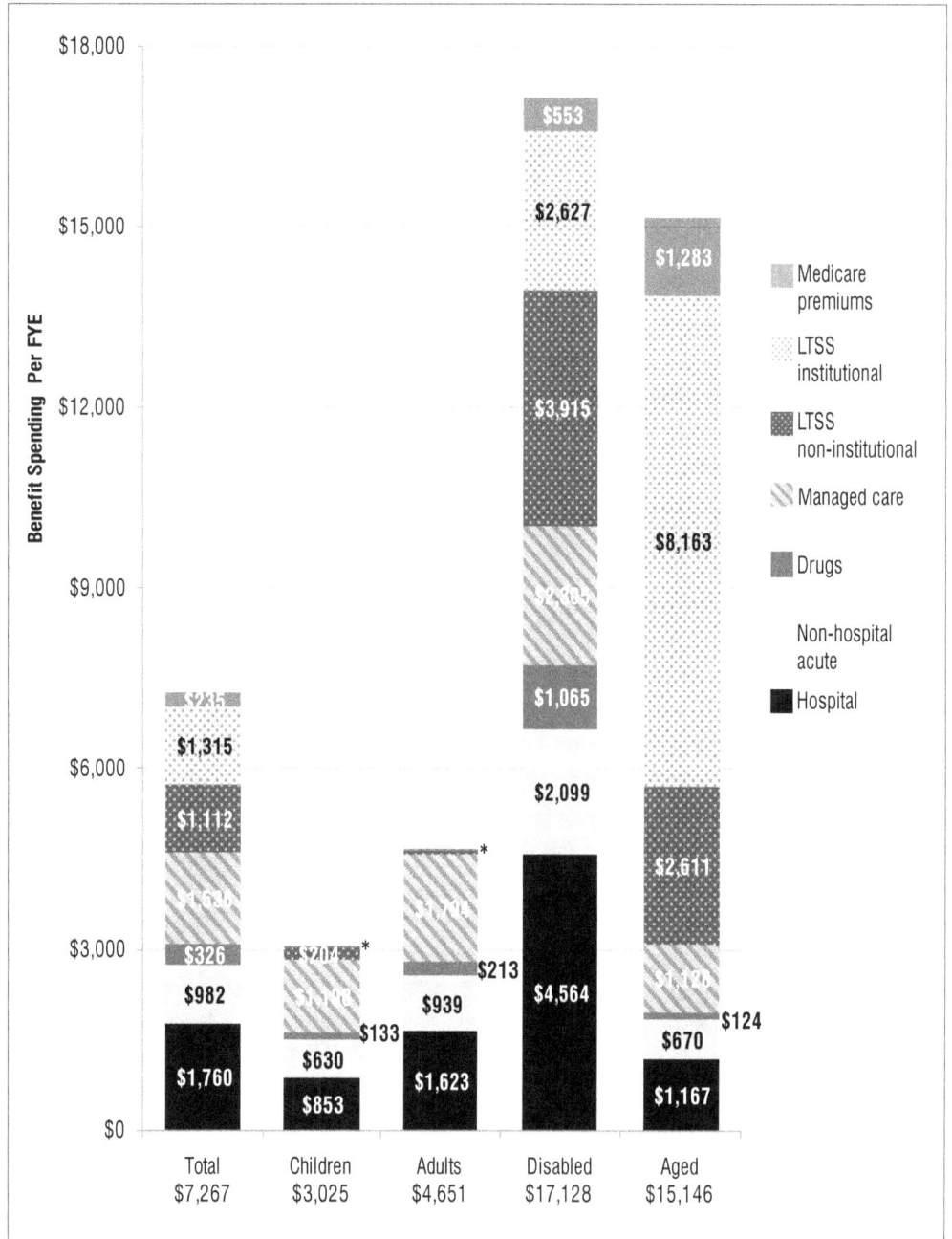

Notes: LTSS = long-term services and supports. Includes federal and state funds. Excludes administrative spending, the territories, and Medicaid-expansion CHIP enrollees. Children and non-aged adults who qualify for Medicaid on the basis of a disability are included in the disabled category. Amounts are fee for service unless otherwise noted. Benefit spending from MSIS data has been adjusted to reflect CMS-64 totals; see Section 4 of MACStats for methodology, including a list of services in each category. Amounts reflect all enrollees, including those with limited benefits; see Table 8 notes for more information.

* Values less than $100 not shown.

Source: MACPAC analysis of Medicaid Statistical Information System (MSIS) annual person summary (APS) data and CMS-64 Financial Management Report (FMR) net expenditure data as of May 2011

FIGURE 5. Distribution of Medicaid Enrollment and Benefit Spending by Users and Non-users of Long-term Services and Supports, FY 2008

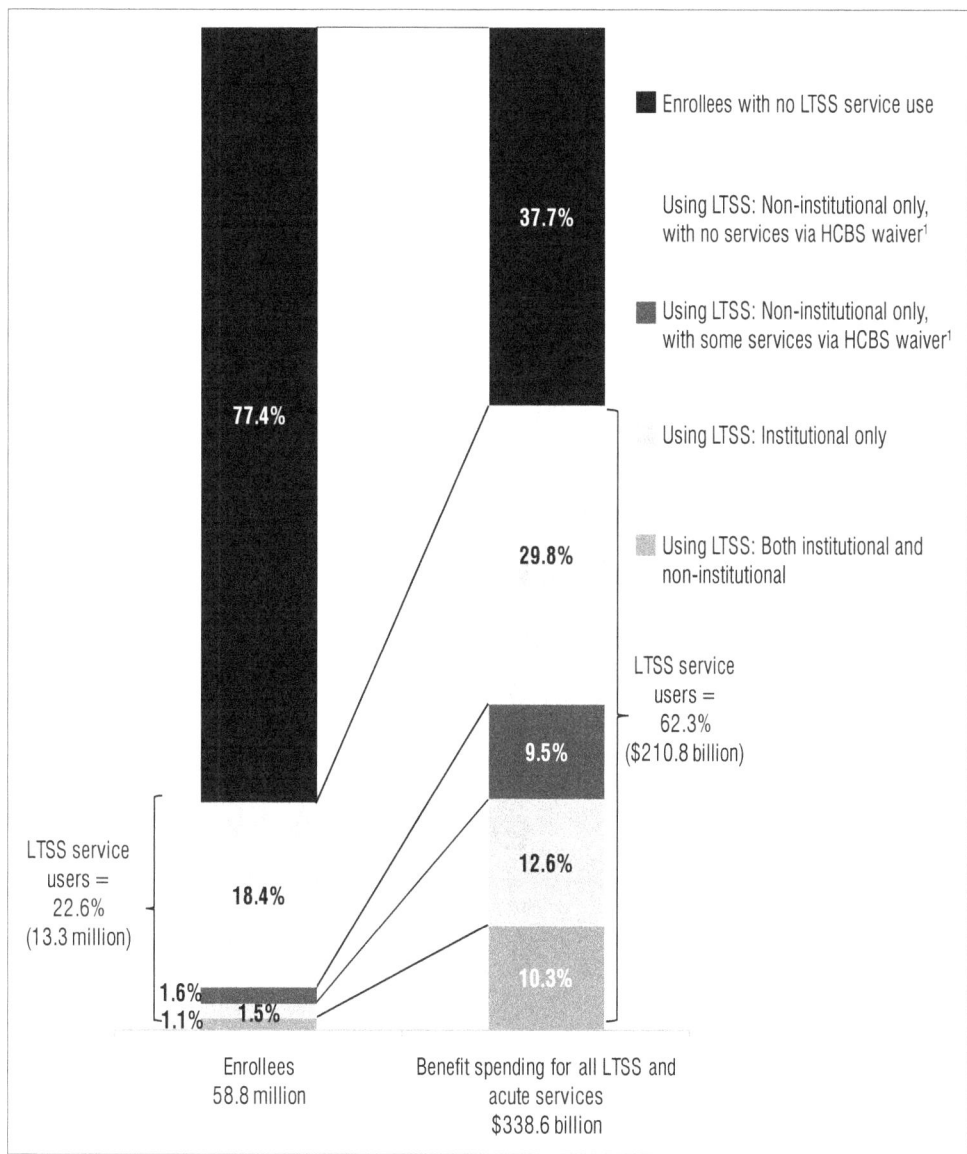

■ Enrollees with no LTSS service use

Using LTSS: Non-institutional only, with no services via HCBS waiver[1]

■ Using LTSS: Non-institutional only, with some services via HCBS waiver[1]

Using LTSS: Institutional only

Using LTSS: Both institutional and non-institutional

LTSS service users = 62.3% ($210.8 billion)

LTSS service users = 22.6% (13.3 million)

77.4%

37.7%

29.8%

9.5%

12.6%

10.3%

18.4%

1.6%

1.1%

1.5%

Enrollees
58.8 million

Benefit spending for all LTSS and acute services
$338.6 billion

Notes: HCBS = home and community-based services, LTSS = long-term services and supports.

Includes federal and state funds. Excludes administrative spending, the territories, and Medicaid-expansion CHIP. Benefit spending from MSIS data has been adjusted to match CMS-64 totals; see Section 4 of MACStats for methodology, including a list of services in each category. LTSS users are defined here as enrollees using at least one LTSS service during the year under a fee-for-service arrangement, regardless of the amount (the data do not allow a breakout of LTSS services delivered through managed care). For example, an enrollee with a short stay in a nursing facility for rehabilitation following a hospital discharge and an enrollee with permanent residence in a nursing facility would both be counted as LTSS users. More refined definitions that take these and other factors into account would produce different results and will be considered in future Commission work.

1 All states have HCBS waivers that provide a range of LTSS for targeted populations of enrollees who require institutional levels of care. Based on a comparison with CMS-372 data (a state-reported source containing aggregate spending and enrollment for HCBS waivers), the number of HCBS waiver enrollees may be underreported in MSIS.

Source: MACPAC analysis of Medicaid Statistical Information System (MSIS) annual person summary (APS) data and CMS-64 Financial Management Report (FMR) net expenditure data from CMS as of May 2011

SECTION 2

MACStats

SECTION 2

MACStats

FIGURE 6. Distribution of Medicaid Benefit Spending by Long-term Services and Supports Use and Service Category, FY 2008

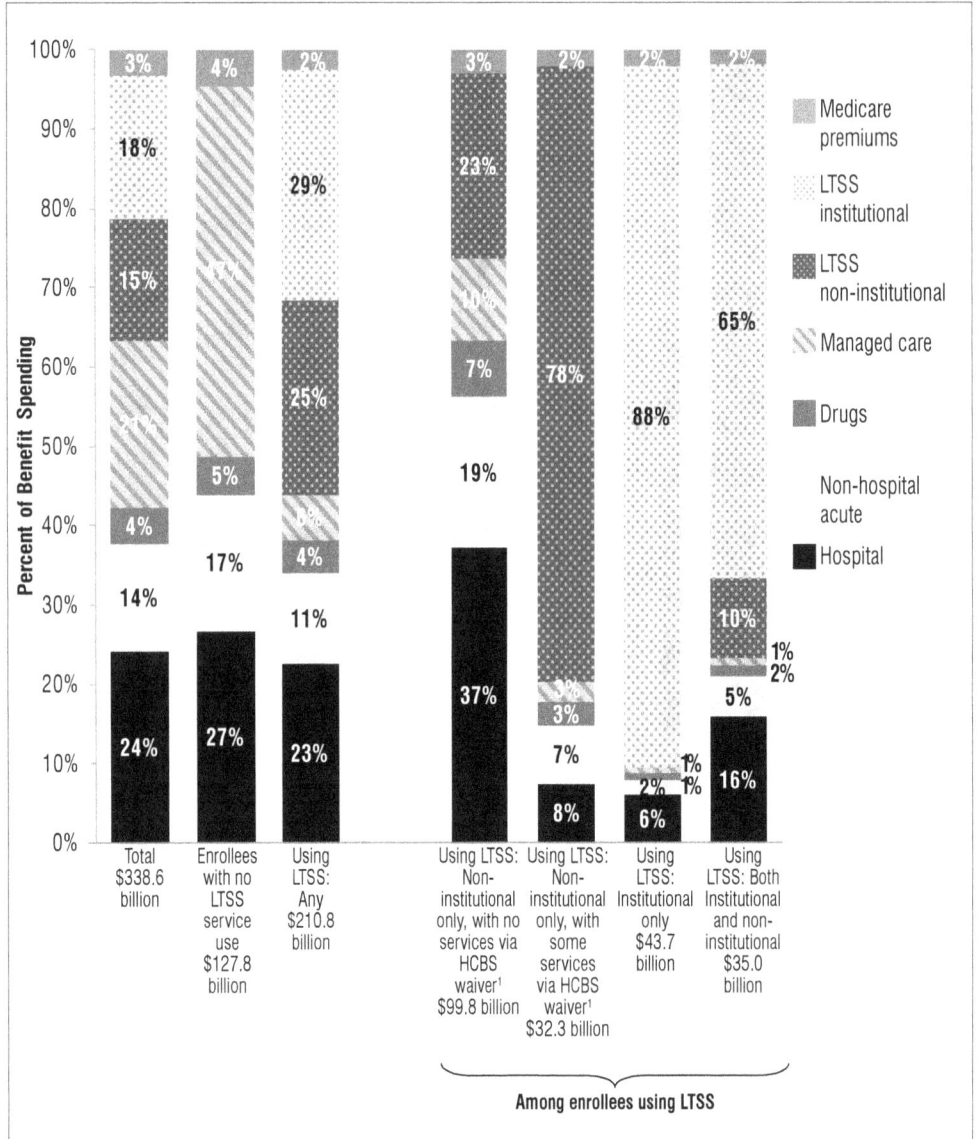

Notes: HCBS = home and community-based services, LTSS = long-term services and supports.

Includes federal and state funds. Excludes administrative spending, the territories, and Medicaid-expansion CHIP. Benefit spending from MSIS data has been adjusted to match CMS-64 totals; see Section 4 of MACStats for methodology, including a list of services in each category. LTSS users are defined here as enrollees using at least one LTSS service during the year under a fee-for-service arrangement, regardless of the amount (the data do not allow a breakout of LTSS services delivered through managed care). For example, an enrollee with a short stay in a nursing facility for rehabilitation following a hospital discharge and an enrollee with permanent residence in a nursing facility would both be counted as LTSS users. More refined definitions that take these and other factors into account would produce different results and will be considered in future Commission work.

1 All states have HCBS waivers that provide a range of LTSS for targeted populations of enrollees who require institutional levels of care. Based on a comparison with CMS-372 data (a state-reported source containing aggregate spending and enrollment for HCBS waivers), the number of HCBS waiver enrollees may be underreported in MSIS.

Source: MACPAC analysis of Medicaid Statistical Information System (MSIS) annual person summary (APS) data and CMS-64 Financial Management Report (FMR) net expenditure data from CMS as of May 2011

FIGURE 7. Medicaid Benefit Spending per Full-year Equivalent (FYE) Enrollee by Long-term Services and Support Use and Service Category, FY 2008

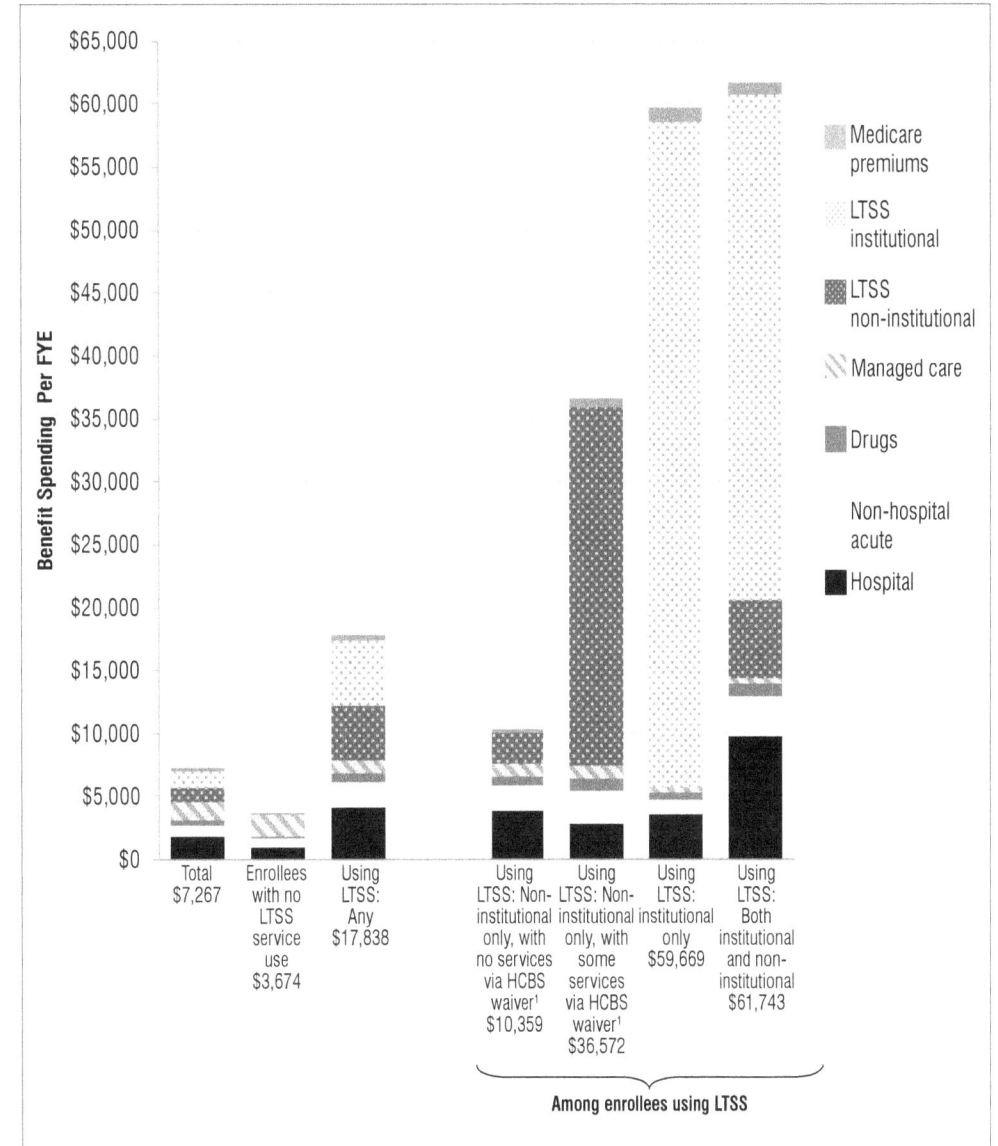

Among enrollees using LTSS

Notes: HCBS = home and community-based services, LTSS = long-term services and supports.

Includes federal and state funds. Excludes administrative spending, the territories, and Medicaid-expansion CHIP enrollees. Benefit spending from MSIS data has been adjusted to match CMS-64 totals; see Section 4 of MACStats for methodology, including a list of services in each category. LTSS users are defined here as enrollees using at least one LTSS service during the year under a fee-for-service arrangement, regardless of the amount (the data do not allow a breakout of LTSS services delivered through managed care). For example, an enrollee with a short stay in a nursing facility for rehabilitation following a hospital discharge and an enrollee with permanent residence in a nursing facility would both be counted as LTSS users. More refined definitions that take these and other factors into account would produce different results and will be considered in future Commission work. Amounts reflect all enrollees, including those with limited benefits; see Table 8 notes for more information.

1 All states have HCBS waivers that provide a range of LTSS for targeted populations of enrollees who require institutional levels of care. Based on a comparison with CMS-372 data (a state-reported source containing aggregate spending and enrollment for HCBS waivers), the number of HCBS waiver enrollees may be underreported in MSIS.

Source: MACPAC analysis of Medicaid Statistical Information System (MSIS) annual person summary (APS) data and CMS-64 Financial Management Report (FMR) net expenditure data from CMS as of May 2011

SECTION

Medicaid Managed Care

The tables in this section provide a state-level supplement to the review of Medicaid managed care in this Report. The national percentage of Medicaid enrollees in managed care (including Medicaid-expansion CHIP) ranges from less than half to 71 percent, depending on the definition of managed care that is used (Table 9). As noted throughout this Report, however, the use of managed care varies widely by state, both in the arrangements used and the populations served. All but two states report using some combination of managed care that involves comprehensive risk-based plans, limited-benefit plans, and primary care case management (PCCM) programs (Tables 9 and 10).

Table 11 shows the share of each of the major Medicaid eligibility groups that is enrolled in managed care, by state. The national percentage of Medicaid enrollees (excluding Medicaid-expansion CHIP) in any form of managed care ranges from 33 percent among aged enrollees to 85 percent among child enrollees. Participation in comprehensive risk-based managed care plans was lowest among the aged and disabled (11 percent and 28 percent, respectively) and highest among adults and children (44 percent and 60 percent). For the total enrollees category, the percentages in any form of managed care and in comprehensive risk-based managed care differ somewhat between Tables 9 and 11; as noted in Section 4, this is due to a variety of differences between MSIS and Medicaid Managed Care Enrollment Report data.

Table 12 shows the share of Medicaid benefit spending for each of the major Medicaid eligibility groups that goes toward payments for managed care. The national percentage of Medicaid benefit spending on any form of managed care ranges from about 7 percent among aged enrollees to nearly 40 percent among non-disabled child and adult enrollees. In states with comprehensive risk-based managed care, these plans make up the majority of managed care spending.

MACStats

SECTION 3

TABLE 9. Percentage of Medicaid Enrollees in Managed Care by State, June 30, 2009

State	Total Medicaid Enrollees	Any managed care[1]	Percentage of Enrollees		
			Comprehensive risk-based or PCCM[2,3]	Comprehensive risk-based[2]	PCCM
Total	**49,450,645**	**71.2%**	**61.5%[4]**	**46.8%**	**14.7%**
Alabama	812,220	66.5	54.6	—	54.6
Alaska	101,702	—	—	—	—
Arizona	1,223,271	89.6	89.6	89.6	—
Arkansas	645,389	79.2	63.7	0.0	63.7
California	6,955,761	52.2	51.9	51.9	—
Colorado	467,556	95.1	14.6	9.8	4.8
Connecticut	455,878	75.2	75.2	75.2	0.0
Delaware	170,562	73.9	68.9	68.9	—
District of Columbia	153,779	97.8	62.8	62.8	—
Florida	2,426,010	66.0	57.3	38.5	18.8
Georgia	1,385,721	92.0	68.3	60.5	7.8
Hawaii	235,203	97.0	97.0	97.0	—
Idaho	198,000	84.1	84.1	—	84.1
Illinois	2,320,700	55.1	55.1	7.7	47.4
Indiana	961,986	74.0	73.9	67.3	6.7
Iowa	397,823	82.9	42.9	0.0	42.9
Kansas	297,290	86.6	55.6	47.5	8.1
Kentucky	768,777	83.0	60.4	20.7	39.7
Louisiana	1,006,842	68.7	72.4	0.0	72.4
Maine	280,148	63.7	63.7	—	63.7
Maryland	787,366	78.7	74.9	74.9	—
Massachusetts	1,227,109	59.6	58.9	35.7	23.2
Michigan	1,629,959	88.8	66.8	66.8	—
Minnesota	675,149	63.1	63.1	63.1	—
Mississippi	673,630	76.1	—	—	—
Missouri	895,077	98.7	44.9	44.9	—
Montana	84,785	66.6	0.5	0.0	0.4
Nebraska	214,699	83.6	34.8	16.8	18.0
Nevada	213,440	83.7	49.8	49.8	—

TABLE 9, Continued

State	Total Medicaid Enrollees	Percentage of Enrollees			
		Any managed care[1]	Comprehensive risk-based or PCCM[2,3]	Comprehensive risk-based[2]	PCCM
New Hampshire	124,498	77.6%	–	–	–
New Jersey	968,598	74.9	74.9%	74.9%	–
New Mexico	464,852	74.2	74.3	74.3	–
New York	4,422,121	66.2	65.5	65.1	0.4%
North Carolina	1,442,396	70.2	69.3	0.0	69.3
North Dakota	60,111	67.6	48.8	0.0	48.8
Ohio	1,951,511	70.4	70.4	70.4	–
Oklahoma	625,546	88.5	65.9	0.0	65.9
Oregon	474,835	88.1	74.0	71.4	2.6
Pennsylvania	1,920,134	82.1	64.0	50.4	13.7
Rhode Island	177,981	62.1	67.7	67.7	–
South Carolina	763,225	100.0	56.6	44.8	11.8
South Dakota	107,196	79.7	79.7	–	79.7
Tennessee	1,230,750	100.0	94.2	94.2	–
Texas	3,343,241	64.6	64.6	42.7	21.9
Utah	238,358	85.9	24.5	–	24.5
Vermont	156,503	87.8	87.8	87.8	–
Virginia	814,820	63.9	64.0	57.3	6.6
Washington	1,103,291	86.0	53.2	52.7	0.4
West Virginia	325,653	46.0	50.5	46.0	4.5
Wisconsin	1,004,704	60.4	57.8	57.8	–
Wyoming	64,489	–	–	–	–

Notes: PCCM = primary care case management. Excludes the territories, unlike other tables and figures in the June 2011 MACStats; includes Medicaid-expansion CHIP enrollees.

– Quantity zero; amounts shown as 0.0 round to less than 0.1 in this table.

1 Any managed care includes comprehensive risk-based plans, limited-benefit plans, and PCCM programs.

2 Comprehensive risk-based managed care includes plans categorized by CMS and states as commercial, Medicaid-only, Health Insuring Organizations (HIOs), and Programs of All-Inclusive Care for the Elderly (PACE). HIOs exist only in California where selected county-authorized health systems serve Medicaid enrollees. PACE combines Medicare and Medicaid financing for qualifying frail elderly dual eligibles. Some states report a larger number of enrollees in these comprehensive risk-based plans than they do for their unduplicated number of enrollees in any form of managed care; it is unclear whether this is a reporting error or whether there were some enrollees participating in more than one comprehensive risk-based plan as of the reporting date (June 30, 2009).

3 Figure is based on the sum of enrollees reported in comprehensive risk-based plans and PCCM programs; it is assumed that individuals are not enrolled in both types of managed care as of the reporting date; but this cannot be verified based on enrollment report data.

4 Unrounded figure is 61.47% and is reported as 61% throughout the text of this Report.

Source: MACPAC analysis of 2009 Medicaid Managed Care Enrollment Report data from CMS, as reported by states

MACStats

SECTION 3

MACStats

SECTION 3

TABLE 10. Number of Managed Care Entities by State and Type, June 30, 2009

State	Comprehensive Risk-based Plans[1]				Limited-benefit Plans[1]			
	Commercial MCO	Medicaid-only MCO	HIO	PACE	PIHP	PAHP	PCCM	Other
Total	**149**	**159**	**4**	**67**	**150**	**60**	**36**	**9**
Alabama	0	0	0	0	2	0	1	0
Alaska	0	0	0	0	0	0	0	0
Arizona	0	29	0	0	1	0	0	0
Arkansas	0	0	0	1	0	1	1	0
California	23	2	4	5	1	13	0	0
Colorado	0	2	0	3	6	0	1	0
Connecticut	1	2	0	0	0	0	1	1
Delaware	0	2	0	0	0	0	0	0
District of Columbia	0	3	0	0	1	1	0	0
Florida	22	5	0	2	26	10	1	3
Georgia	0	3	0	0	0	1	1	0
Hawaii	4	1	0	1	0	0	0	0
Idaho	0	0	0	0	0	2	1	1
Illinois	1	2	0	0	0	0	1	0
Indiana	4	1	0	0	0	0	2	0
Iowa	0	0	0	1	1	0	1	0
Kansas	0	2	0	2	1	1	1	0
Kentucky	0	1	0	0	0	1	1	0
Louisiana	0	0	0	1	0	1	1	0
Maine	0	0	0	0	0	0	1	0
Maryland	0	7	0	1	0	5	0	0
Massachusetts	2	2	0	6	1	0	1	0
Michigan	0	14	0	4	18	0	0	0
Minnesota	6	3	0	0	0	0	0	0
Mississippi	0	0	0	0	0	1	0	0
Missouri	0	6	0	1	0	1	1	0
Montana	0	0	0	1	0	1	1	0
Nebraska	1	0	0	0	0	0	1	1

TABLE 10, Continued

State	Comprehensive Risk-based Plans[1]					Limited-benefit Plans[1]				
	Commercial MCO	Medicaid-only MCO	HIO	PACE	PIHP	PAHP	PCCM	Other		
Nevada	1	1	0	0	0	1	0	0		
New Hampshire	0	0	0	0	0	1	0	0		
New Jersey	2	3	0	2	0	0	0	0		
New Mexico	5	1	0	1	1	0	0	1		
New York	21	13	0	5	17	0	4	1		
North Carolina	0	0	0	2	1	0	2	0		
North Dakota	0	0	0	1	0	1	1	0		
Ohio	0	7	0	2	0	0	0	0		
Oklahoma	0	0	0	1	0	1	2	0		
Oregon	2	13	0	1	9	8	1	0		
Pennsylvania	11	0	0	10	38	2	1	0		
Rhode Island	2	1	0	1	0	1	0	0		
South Carolina	0	6	0	2	0	3	1	0		
South Dakota	0	0	0	0	0	0	1	0		
Tennessee	0	6	0	1	2	0	0	2		
Texas	6	13	0	2	1	1	1	0		
Utah	0	0	0	0	11	1	1	0		
Vermont	0	1	0	1	0	0	0	0		
Virginia	3	2	0	4	0	1	1	0		
Washington	8	0	0	1	1	1	1	0		
West Virginia	3	0	0	0	0	0	1	0		
Wisconsin	21	5	0	1	11	0	0	0		
Wyoming	0	0	0	0	0	0	0	0		

Notes: HIO = Health Insuring Organization; MCO = managed care organization; PACE = Program of All-Inclusive Care for the Elderly; PAHP = prepaid ambulatory health plan; PIHP = prepaid inpatient health plan; PCCM = primary care case management. Excludes the territories.

Comprehensive risk-based managed care includes plans categorized by CMS and states as commercial, Medicaid-only, Health Insuring Organizations (HIOs), and Programs of All-Inclusive Care for the Elderly (PACE). HIOs exist only in California where selected county-authorized health systems serve Medicaid enrollees. PACE combines Medicare and Medicaid financing for qualifying frail elderly dual eligibles. In the data reporting instructions provided by CMS to states, commercial plans are those that provide comprehensive services to both Medicaid and commercial and/or Medicare enrollees; Medicaid-only plans are those that provide comprehensive services to only Medicaid enrollees, not to commercial or Medicare enrollees. Based on an examination of plan names, it appears that states differ in their categorizations; for example, plans that operate in different states but are affiliated with the same parent company may be reported as commercial in one state and Medicaid-only in another.

1 These terms are used throughout the Report to categorize the various plan types shown; see Annex C for additional plan definitions.

Source: 2009 Medicaid Managed Care Enrollment Report data from CMS, as reported by states

MACStats

SECTION 3

MACStats

SECTION 3

TABLE 11. Percentage of Medicaid Enrollees in Managed Care by State and Eligibility Group, FY 2008

	Percentage of Enrollees									
	Any managed care					Comprehensive risk-based managed care				
State	Total	Children	Adults	Disabled	Aged	Total	Children	Adults	Disabled	Aged
Total	**68.3%**	**84.6%**	**57.1%**	**58.4%**	**32.9%**	**46.0%**	**60.0%**	**43.8%**	**27.9%**	**10.9%**
Alabama	67.2	97.2	21.0	62.0	17.2	2.8	0.0	0.0	5.8	12.6
Alaska	–	–	–	–	–	–	–	–	–	–
Arizona	87.3	94.6	79.2	95.6	70.8	80.8	88.3	72.0	88.7	67.4
Arkansas	59.9	85.1	24.2	54.5	4.4	–	–	–	–	–
California	58.1	77.1	26.7	93.8	85.9	37.3	62.0	22.0	23.9	15.0
Colorado	90.4	95.2	84.3	85.7	79.6	19.9	24.6	12.3	16.1	11.1
Connecticut	59.7	81.4	72.4	0.9	0.0	59.7	81.4	72.4	0.9	0.0
Delaware	87.5	97.0	87.3	78.1	46.4	73.0	85.9	78.8	48.6	2.6
District of Columbia	64.8	89.9	84.6	11.6	0.2	64.8	89.9	84.6	11.6	0.2
Florida	70.3	88.9	75.5	52.7	12.4	63.1	82.6	57.0	49.8	11.8
Georgia	88.4	95.8	89.3	81.5	48.0	67.2	90.8	83.9	2.8	0.0
Hawaii	75.9	97.1	93.4	12.8	1.3	75.9	97.1	93.4	12.7	1.3
Idaho	89.8	97.5	92.5	79.9	49.6	0.2	0.1	0.1	0.6	0.5
Illinois	67.5	83.3	71.4	30.3	5.9	7.4	10.1	7.7	0.1	0.1
Indiana	77.1	90.7	85.0	48.8	14.5	69.8	89.2	85.0	14.0	0.1
Iowa	75.5	94.6	57.7	92.4	4.5	1.5	2.3	1.5	0.1	0.0
Kansas	85.4	94.6	89.2	79.2	40.7	85.4	94.6	89.2	79.2	40.7
Kentucky	88.6	95.0	96.9	84.7	51.3	19.0	23.6	20.3	15.2	4.6
Louisiana	62.6	88.7	44.1	41.4	1.4	0.0	–	–	0.0	0.1
Maine	–	–	–	–	–	–	–	–	–	–
Maryland	67.0	93.2	46.2	53.2	0.8	67.0	93.2	46.2	53.2	0.8
Massachusetts	54.6	82.8	73.7	29.6	10.1	31.2	58.6	37.1	10.1	8.8
Michigan	70.4	86.5	63.9	53.4	3.0	66.7	81.2	62.7	50.6	2.5
Minnesota	69.2	87.1	71.4	12.2	61.0	69.2	87.1	71.4	12.2	61.0
Mississippi	–	–	–	–	–	–	–	–	–	–
Missouri	73.1	66.7	59.5	96.2	91.3	46.9	66.6	59.2	1.8	0.0
Montana	48.7	62.7	36.9	42.1	0.6	–	–	–	–	–
Nebraska	36.9	46.5	42.0	19.9	2.9	17.5	21.9	20.3	9.7	1.3
Nevada	87.9	95.9	87.6	76.2	59.9	54.9	73.9	68.4	1.7	0.0
New Hampshire	–	–	–	–	–	–	–	–	–	–
New Jersey	70.6	92.7	80.9	42.6	8.2	70.6	92.7	80.9	42.6	8.2

TABLE 11, Continued

State	Any managed care					Comprehensive risk-based managed care				
	Total	Children	Adults	Disabled	Aged	Total	Children	Adults	Disabled	Aged
New Mexico	66.8%	79.3%	56.6%	50.4%	3.4%	66.7%	79.2%	56.5%	50.0%	3.4%
New York	66.1	79.6	75.9	39.8	12.8	66.1	79.6	75.9	39.8	12.8
North Carolina	71.0	91.5	62.2	54.2	16.2	0.0	–	–	0.0	0.0
North Dakota	52.8	72.4	74.8	1.6	0.0	–	–	–	–	–
Ohio	71.3	87.7	88.5	40.3	6.8	71.3	87.7	88.5	40.3	6.8
Oklahoma	86.1	96.1	58.7	86.4	82.1	–	–	–	–	–
Oregon	86.6	92.8	83.1	82.4	70.7	70.6	80.1	72.5	58.1	37.4
Pennsylvania	87.8	95.1	86.1	92.1	49.7	59.6	73.0	65.1	53.1	7.1
Rhode Island	61.0	89.6	90.4	11.4	0.2	61.0	89.6	90.4	11.4	0.2
South Carolina	89.8	98.6	69.8	94.2	85.3	30.6	43.5	26.0	16.6	0.0
South Dakota	100.0	100.0	100.0	100.0	100.0	–	–	–	–	–
Tennessee	93.0	97.0	97.4	92.0	53.9	92.9	96.9	97.4	91.7	53.9
Texas	71.7	90.3	51.5	45.4	19.4	46.8	59.8	34.8	22.4	14.9
Utah	73.1	87.6	44.1	74.0	73.3	0.3	0.1	–	1.6	0.2
Vermont	–†	–†	–†	–†	–†	–†	–†	–†	–†	–†
Virginia	66.6	83.9	72.4	43.8	16.3	59.6	78.1	67.2	35.9	2.8
Washington	67.0	84.7	55.8	47.3	12.8	65.8	84.1	55.3	42.6	12.1
West Virginia	55.3	90.1	78.9	3.1	0.0	48.9	79.9	70.9	1.7	0.0
Wisconsin	54.1	76.3	58.3	27.0	10.4	51.5	75.0	57.4	22.3	2.9
Wyoming	–	–	–	–	–	–	–	–	–	–

Percentage of Enrollees

Notes: Excludes the territories and Medicaid-expansion CHIP enrollees. Children and adults under age 65 who qualify for Medicaid on the basis of a disability are included in the disabled category. Any managed care includes comprehensive risk-based plans, limited-benefit plans, and primary care case management programs. Enrollees are counted as participating in managed care if they were enrolled during the fiscal year and at least one managed care payment was made on their behalf during the fiscal year; this method underestimates participation somewhat because it does not capture enrollees who entered managed care late in the year but for whom a payment was not made until the following fiscal year.

Figures shown here may differ from Table 9, which uses Medicaid Managed Care Enrollment Report data. Reasons for differences include differing time periods (ever in FY 2008 for MSIS), state reporting anomalies (e.g., some states report a very small number of comprehensive risk-based enrollees in MSIS who may be miscategorized), and Medicaid-expansion CHIP enrollees (excluded here but included in Table 9). Although the enrollment report used for Table 9 is a commonly cited source, it does not provide information on the characteristics of enrollees in managed care (e.g., eligibility group) or their spending and non-managed care service use. MSIS data are used here to provide this additional level of detail.

– Quantity zero; amounts shown as 0.0 round to less than 0.1 in this table.

† Due to large differences in the way managed care spending is reported by Vermont in CMS-64 and MSIS data, managed care enrollment (which, for this table, is based on the presence of managed care spending in MSIS for a given enrollee) is not reported here.

Source: MACPAC analysis of Medicaid Statistical Information System (MSIS) annual person summary (APS) data from CMS as of May 2011

Updated on July 25, 2011. Table 11 reflects the addition of a clarifying footnote after the Report's publication.

SECTION 3

MACStats

MACStats

TABLE 12. Percentage of Medicaid Benefit Spending on Managed Care by State and Eligibility Group, FY 2008

	Percentage of Benefit Spending									
	Any managed care					Comprehensive risk-based managed care				
State	Total	Children	Adults	Disabled	Aged	Total	Children	Adults	Disabled	Aged
Total	**21.1%**	**39.6%**	**38.6%**	**13.5%**	**7.4%**	**18.2%**	**34.5%**	**34.8%**	**10.9%**	**6.4%**
Alabama	15.3	40.3	6.5	8.7	0.5	0.1	0.0	0.0	0.1	0.2
Alaska	–	–	–	–	–	–	–	–	–	–
Arizona	84.0	86.0	83.0	84.2	81.5	70.0	64.6	65.4	78.1	74.7
Arkansas	0.4	1.3	0.4	0.2	0.0	–	–	–	–	–
California	15.5	39.1	13.7	8.9	12.0	13.9	35.5	12.5	8.1	10.0
Colorado	12.5	21.3	7.7	11.3	8.6	5.9	7.8	4.1	4.4	7.7
Connecticut	13.5	45.8	51.3	0.1	0.0	13.5	45.8	51.3	0.1	0.0
Delaware	39.0	47.0	70.3	26.3	1.0	38.2	45.1	69.3	26.0	0.8
District of Columbia	19.6	40.7	51.7	8.5	0.0	19.6	40.7	51.7	8.5	0.0
Florida	16.8	31.0	16.6	14.2	9.7	15.3	28.2	16.2	12.4	9.6
Georgia	30.4	67.4	65.6	1.6	0.7	29.1	65.1	64.8	0.3	0.0
Hawaii	29.2	72.7	74.5	1.5	0.2	28.4	68.0	74.4	1.5	0.2
Idaho	3.0	9.0	2.8	0.6	0.9	0.0	0.0	0.0	0.0	0.0
Illinois	2.0	4.7	4.8	0.1	0.3	1.3	3.1	3.4	0.0	0.2
Indiana	18.4	50.4	62.7	2.8	0.0	18.4	50.3	62.7	2.7	0.0
Iowa	4.5	8.5	6.4	4.5	0.1	0.3	0.9	0.9	0.0	0.0
Kansas	23.0	59.0	72.5	9.6	2.1	22.9	58.9	72.5	9.6	2.1
Kentucky	16.6	27.8	21.2	15.6	1.5	15.1	24.0	19.5	14.8	1.2
Louisiana	0.1	0.2	0.0	0.0	0.0	0.0	–	–	0.0	0.0
Maine	–	–	–	–	–	–	–	–	–	–
Maryland	32.1	52.6	66.9	27.4	0.5	32.1	52.6	66.8	27.4	0.5
Massachusetts	26.0	49.4	39.7	17.3	14.4	22.1	45.4	30.7	13.2	14.3
Michigan	43.0	54.9	62.9	47.2	3.9	37.3	52.5	54.7	39.4	1.3
Minnesota	30.4	67.7	67.9	3.8	36.1	30.4	67.7	67.9	3.9	36.1
Mississippi	–	–	–	–	–	–	–	–	–	–
Missouri	14.8	39.8	37.4	0.7	1.1	14.3	39.8	37.4	0.1	0.0
Montana	0.4	1.2	0.3	0.2	0.0	–	–	–	–	–

TABLE 12, Continued

State	Any managed care					Comprehensive risk-based managed care				
	Total	Children	Adults	Disabled	Aged	Total	Children	Adults	Disabled	Aged
Nebraska	5.7%	10.8%	14.4%	3.6%	0.7%	5.6%	10.6%	14.3%	3.6%	0.7%
Nevada	13.9	33.6	38.2	0.4	0.3	13.2	32.0	37.2	0.1	0.0
New Hampshire	–	–	–	–	–	–	–	–	–	–
New Jersey	16.2	43.5	54.9	8.0	1.4	16.2	43.5	54.9	8.0	1.4
New Mexico	47.2	69.2	58.7	36.3	3.6	39.4	55.4	54.7	29.9	3.5
New York	16.5	37.9	40.1	6.8	8.1	16.5	37.8	40.1	6.8	8.1
North Carolina	1.2	1.9	0.5	1.5	0.2	0.0	–	–	0.0	0.0
North Dakota	0.3	1.5	0.9	0.0	0.0	–	–	–	–	–
Ohio	32.9	75.3	80.5	23.6	3.6	32.9	75.3	80.5	23.6	3.6
Oklahoma	4.6	10.2	3.9	2.7	1.6	–	–	–	–	–
Oregon	36.7	53.5	63.1	32.6	9.7	28.5	37.3	56.1	24.3	8.1
Pennsylvania	41.4	73.5	66.8	47.0	5.6	27.0	50.6	48.4	29.1	2.8
Rhode Island	19.3	49.9	73.0	4.9	0.0	19.3	49.8	73.0	4.9	0.0
South Carolina	8.0	15.2	11.3	5.7	1.6	6.7	12.6	10.4	5.1	0.0
South Dakota	0.2	0.6	0.2	0.1	0.1	–	–	–	–	–
Tennessee	48.4	72.1	73.1	41.0	9.7	35.3	55.7	59.5	25.7	8.8
Texas	18.3	32.2	21.5	8.9	8.9	18.0	31.8	21.4	8.5	8.9
Utah	11.1	7.5	4.3	17.8	4.9	0.7	0.3	–	1.4	0.1
Vermont	78.2	–	–	–	–	–	–	–	–	–
Virginia	23.5	38.3	50.1	19.3	2.4	23.4	38.3	50.1	19.3	2.4
Washington	24.1	65.6	58.7	1.7	1.5	24.1	65.6	58.7	1.7	1.5
West Virginia	11.7	37.8	44.8	0.2	0.0	11.7	37.7	44.8	0.2	0.0
Wisconsin	26.2	44.7	51.0	16.5	20.2	17.1	41.6	49.0	8.7	3.0
Wyoming	–	–	–	–	–	–	–	–	–	–

Note: Includes federal and state funds. Excludes administrative spending, the territories, and Medicaid-expansion CHIP enrollees. Children and non-aged adults who qualify for Medicaid on the basis of a disability are included in the disabled category. Benefit spending from MSIS data has been adjusted to match CMS-64 totals; see Section 4 of MACStats for methodology. Any managed care includes comprehensive risk-based plans, limited-benefit plans, and primary care case management programs.

– Quantity zero; amounts shown as 0.0 round to less than 0.1 in this table.

1 Due to large differences in the way managed care spending is reported by Vermont in CMS-64 and MSIS data, benefit spending based on MACPAC's adjustment methodology is not reported at a level lower than total Medicaid managed care.

Source: MACPAC analysis of Medicaid Statistical Information System (MSIS) annual person summary (APS) data and CMS-64 Financial Management Report (FMR) net expenditure data from CMS as of May 2011

SECTION 3

MACStats

SECTION

Technical Guide to the June 2011 MACStats

This section provides supplemental information to accompany the tables and figures in Sections 1, 2, and 3 of MACStats. It describes key issues to be aware of when interpreting the data, comparing numbers across tables and figures, or reconciling findings with data from other sources.

Guide to Interpreting Medicaid and CHIP Numbers

As described in MACPAC's March 2011 Report, there are several reasons why estimates of Medicaid and CHIP enrollment and spending may vary.[34] These issues are noted here in relation to the tables and figures in the June 2011 of MACStats. In addition, MACPAC has made certain adjustments to spending data in MACStats that are described in detail later in this section.

Data Sources

Medicaid and CHIP enrollment and spending numbers are available from administrative data, which states and the federal government compile in the course of administering the programs. The latest year of available data differs, depending on the source. The administrative data used in this edition of MACStats include the following, which are submitted to CMS by states:

- Form CMS-64 for state-level Medicaid spending, as used throughout MACStats;

- The Medicaid Statistical Information System (MSIS) for person-level detail, as used throughout MACStats[35]; and

---

[34] See MACPAC, *Report to the Congress on Medicaid and CHIP: March 2011* (Washington, DC: MACPAC, 2001): 75-77. http://www.macpac.gov/reports/ MACPAC_March2011_web.pdf.

[35] MACPAC has adjusted benefit spending from MSIS to match CMS-64 totals; see discussion later in Section 4 for details.

▶ Medicaid managed care enrollment reports, as used in Tables 9 and 10.

Additional information is available from some nationally representative surveys based on interviews of individuals. The survey data used in Tables 3A–5C are from HHS's National Health Interview Survey (NHIS).

Enrollment Period Examined

The number of individuals enrolled at a particular point during the year will be smaller than the number ever enrolled during the year. Point-in-time data may also be referred to as average monthly enrollment or full-year equivalent enrollment.[36] Full-year equivalent enrollment is often used for budget analyses, such as those by CMS's Office of the Actuary, and when comparing enrollment and expenditure numbers, as in Figure 1. Per enrollee spending levels based on full-year equivalents (Table 8) ensure that amounts are not biased by individuals' transitions in and out of Medicaid coverage during the year.

Enrollees versus Beneficiaries

Depending on the data source and the year in question, CMS may refer to individuals in Medicaid as enrollees or eligibles—or as beneficiaries, recipients, or persons served. For this version of MACStats and the topics examined in this report, it is important to recognize how individuals and spending are counted and described in administrative data sources provided by CMS:

▶ **Enrollees or eligibles**—CMS refers to individuals who are eligible for and enrolled in Medicaid or CHIP as either enrollees or eligibles.

▶ **Beneficiaries, recipients, or persons served**—Enrollees who receive covered services or for whom Medicaid or CHIP payments are made (including managed care payments) are generally referred to as beneficiaries, recipients, or persons served.[37]

▶ **Medicaid-expansion CHIP**—Depending on the data source, Medicaid enrollment and spending figures may include both Medicaid enrollees funded with Medicaid dollars and Medicaid-expansion CHIP enrollees funded with CHIP dollars.

Prior to FY 1990, CMS did not track the number of Medicaid enrollees—only beneficiaries. For some historical numbers, CMS has estimated the number of enrollees prior to 1990 (Figure 1).

Prior to FY 1998, individuals were not counted as beneficiaries if managed care payments were the only Medicaid payments made on their behalf. Beginning in FY 1998, however, Medicaid managed care enrollees with no fee-for-service (FFS) spending were also counted as beneficiaries, which had a large impact on the numbers (Table 1).[38]

The following example illustrates the difference in these terms. In FY 2008, there were 9.7 million disabled Medicaid *enrollees* (Table 6). However, there were 8.7 million disabled *beneficiaries*—that is, during FY 2008, a Medicaid fee for service or

---

[36] Average monthly enrollment takes the state-submitted monthly enrollment numbers (i.e., 12 separate point-in-time enrollment numbers) and averages them over the 12-month period. It produces the same result as full-year equivalent enrollment or person-years, which is the sum of total person-months for the year divided by 12.

[37] See, for example, CMS, Brief Summaries and Glossary in *Health Care Financing Review 2010 Statistical Supplement*, https://www.cms.gov/MedicareMedicaidStatSupp/LT/list.asp.

[38] In a given year, it is possible that no payments were made for an enrollee who used no Medicaid services and was not enrolled in managed care. However, if the individual were enrolled in managed care, the state would make capitated Medicaid payments to the plan on behalf of the individual, even if no health care services were used. Therefore, all managed care enrollees are now counted as beneficiaries, whether or not they use any health services.

managed care capitation payment was made on their behalf (Table 1).[39] Generally, the number of beneficiaries will approach the number of enrollees as more of these individuals use Medicaid-covered services or are enrolled in managed care.[40]

Institutionalized and Limited-benefit Enrollees

Administrative Medicaid data include those who were in institutions such as nursing homes, as well as individuals who received only limited benefits (for example, only coverage for emergency services). Survey data tend to exclude such individuals from counts of coverage; the NHIS estimates in Tables 3A-5C do not include the institutionalized.

CHIP Enrollees

Medicaid-expansion CHIP enrollees are children who are entitled to the covered services of the state Medicaid program but are generally funded with CHIP dollars. We exclude these children from Medicaid analyses where possible, but in some cases data sources do not allow Medicaid-expansion CHIP enrollees to be broken out separately (e.g., Table 9 includes these enrollees, while nearly all other tables and figures in MACStats exclude them).

Medicaid Eligibility for Persons with Disabilities

The following briefly describes Medicaid eligibility for persons with disabilities. The purpose of this section is to provide context for interpreting the health characteristics and Medicaid enrollment, service use and expenditures of the disabled populations in the tables and figures in MACStats and the managed care sections of this Report.

For purposes of program enrollment and spending data, the Medicaid program's classification of "disabled" generally refers to Medicaid enrollees under age 65 who qualify for Medicaid on the basis of a disability. Medicaid enrollees who qualify for coverage due to a disability have conditions that include physical impairments and limitations (e.g., quadriplegia), intellectual or developmental impairments (e.g., mental retardation, cerebral palsy), and severe mental and emotional conditions, including mental illness (e.g., schizophrenia).

- For most enrollees with disabilities, qualifying on the basis of a disability means qualifying for benefits under the federal Supplemental Security Income (SSI) program.[41]

- Working individuals with disabilities with incomes too high to qualify for SSI may qualify for Medicaid through other disability-related provisions that would lead them to be classified as disabled in most Medicaid program statistics, including Medicaid buy-in programs, described later in this section; many of these individuals receive Social Security Disability Insurance (SSDI) benefits.

SECTION 4

MACStats

---

[39] Some individuals who are counted as beneficiaries in CMS data for a particular fiscal year were not enrolled in Medicaid during that year; they are individuals who were enrolled and received services in a prior year but for whom a lagged payment was made in the following year. These individuals usually have an "unknown" basis of eligibility in CMS data.

[40] Analyses of growth in the number of Medicaid beneficiaries will sometimes refer to "enrollment growth" in a generic sense.

[41] Eleven states use different Medicaid eligibility rules from the federal SSI program. Known as "209(b) states," these states can use more restrictive eligibility criteria (financial and non-financial) for Medicaid eligibility than the federal SSI program, as long as the Medicaid rules are no more restrictive than the rules the state had in place in 1972 when SSI was enacted.

SECTION 4

MACStats

▶ Individuals with disabilities—or conditions that might be considered disabling—who have incomes too high to qualify for SSI but still have low incomes or high medical expenses may also be covered at state option through poverty level, medically needy, special income level, and other eligibility pathways (March 2011 MACStats Table 11). Some of these pathways are specific to people who require an institutional level of care, but services may be provided in the community (e.g., under a 1915(c) home and community-based services (HCBS) waiver) or in a nursing or other facility depending on the state and the individual's circumstances.[42] The extent to which individuals under age 65 who qualify for Medicaid through one of these pathways are classified as disabled in program statistics may vary based on state practices.

▶ Individuals with disabilities may also qualify for Medicaid under provisions that are unrelated to disability status—for example, as a child in foster care or as the low-income parent of a dependent child.

Of the 58.8 million people enrolled in Medicaid in FY 2008, 9.7 million (16.5 percent) were nonelderly individuals who qualified for Medicaid benefits on the basis of a disability (Table 6), including approximately 1.4 million individuals under age 19. Approximately 4 million of these individuals are also eligible for Medicare, and are known as dual eligibles.[43]

Qualifying for SSI and Medicaid

SSI provides cash assistance to low-income people who are aged, blind, or disabled and meet certain income and resource requirements. The SSI monthly income standard for 2011 is $674 (75 percent of the federal poverty limit, or FPL) for an individual and $1,011 (83 percent FPL) for a couple. The asset standard is $2,000 and $3,000 for individuals and couples, respectively.

To meet the definition of disability for SSI, an adult must have a medically determinable physical or mental impairment (or multiple impairments) that prevents the individual from being engaged in substantial gainful activity (SGA) (§1614(a)(3)(A) of the Social Security Act). The impairment must be expected to last at least 12 months. A person who is earning more than a certain monthly amount (net of impairment-related work expenses) is considered to be engaging in substantial gainful activity. The monthly SGA amount for 2011 is $1,640 for blind individuals and $1,000 for non-blind individuals.

Children under age 18 meet SSI's disability definition if they have a medically determinable physical or mental impairment that results in "marked and severe functional limitations" (§1614(a)(3)(C)(i) of the Social Security Act). Again, the impairment must be expected to last for at least 12 months. A child may be eligible for SSI as early as the date of birth. At age 18 the Social Security Administration (SSA) will reevaluate the individual's impairments based on the definition of disability for adults.

---

[42] HCBS waivers target populations that are "at risk of institutional care," including the frail elderly, individuals with physical disabilities, individuals with mental retardation and developmental disabilities, medically fragile or technology-dependent children, individuals with HIV/AIDS, and individuals with traumatic brain and spinal cord injury.

[43] This includes "partial" dual eligible enrollees who receive only limited Medicaid benefits (i.e., financial assistance for Medicare premiums, deductibles and cost sharing) known as Qualified Medicare Beneficiaries (QMBs), Specified Low-Income Medicare Beneficiaries (SLMBs), and Qualifying Individuals (QIs).

In 39 states and the District of Columbia, individuals who receive cash assistance under SSI on the basis of a disability are automatically eligible for Medicaid. In 32 of these states the SSI application is also the Medicaid application, and Medicaid eligibility starts the same month as SSI eligibility, based on SSA's determination of disability. Seven states (Alaska, Idaho, Kansas, Nebraska, Nevada, Oregon, and Utah) use the same rules to decide eligibility for Medicaid that SSA uses for SSI, but require the filing of a separate application. The state makes the final eligibility determination.

Eleven states (Connecticut, Hawaii, Illinois, Indiana, Minnesota, Missouri, New Hampshire, North Dakota, Ohio, Oklahoma, and Virginia) may use Medicaid eligibility rules that are more restrictive than the federal SSI program. These states are known as 209(b) states. In 209(b) states, both the financial and non-financial eligibility criteria for Medicaid eligibility determination can be more restrictive than the federal SSI program as long as the Medicaid rules are no more restrictive than the rules the state had in place in 1972 when the SSI program was enacted.

Medicaid and the Working Disabled

Basing the definition of disability on an individual's work status has the potential to create a disincentive for individuals to return to work. To address this issue, Medicaid includes mandatory (e.g., for Qualified Severely Impaired Individuals) and optional (e.g., Medicaid buy-in programs) provisions that allow certain individuals with disabilities to work and retain Medicaid eligibility. As of 2009, over 150,000 individuals were enrolled in Medicaid coverage under Medicaid optional buy-in programs for the working disabled.[44]

Qualified Severely Impaired Individuals

Some individuals with disabilities are able to work, but only when they have medical coverage for their condition. Under Section 1905(q) of the Social Security Act, states must continue Medicaid eligibility for individuals under age 65 who (1) continue to have a disabling physical or mental impairment on the basis of which they were found to be disabled, (2) need Medicaid coverage in order to continue working, (3) would lose SSI and Medicaid because their earnings exceed the substantial gainful activity monthly standard, and (4) continue to meet other requirements for Medicaid and SSI. These individuals are entitled to receive Medicaid after the loss of SSI due to earnings until they reach an income level considered sufficient by SSA for them to purchase a "reasonable equivalent" of SSI benefits, Medicaid benefits, and publicly funded attendant care services.

Medicaid Buy-In Programs

There are several other options for individuals who want to return to work without losing their Medicaid benefits. The Balanced Budget Act of 1997 (BBA, P.L. 105-33) created a state option to permit workers with disabilities to buy into Medicaid; states may charge these individuals a monthly premium or other cost sharing based on income. To qualify, individuals must:

- meet the definition of disabled under the Social Security Act and be eligible for SSI payments if not for earnings;

- have earnings that exceed the maximum amount permitted for the maintenance of Medicaid benefits as a qualified severely impaired individual; and

---

[44] M. Kehn et al., Appendix B-14 in A *Government Performance and Results (GPRA) report: The status of the Medicaid Infrastructure Grants Program as of 12/31/09* (Washington, DC: Mathematica Policy Research Inc., 2010).

SECTION 4

MACStats

▸ be in a family whose net income is less than 250 percent of the FPL for its size. For a family of three in 2011 this would be $3,860 a month. States may use less restrictive methodologies to increase the income and resource thresholds.

The Ticket to Work and Work Incentives Improvement Act of 1999 (TWWIIA, P.L.106-170) created two additional Medicaid buy-in options for the working disabled.

▸ Section 1902(a)(10)(A)(ii)(XV) of the Social Security Act allows states to offer a buy-in to working age individuals (age 18-64) who would be eligible, except for earnings, for SSI. States can set eligibility limits on assets and earned and unearned income and set the methodologies for determining income and resources. States can impose premiums or other cost sharing based on income.

▸ Section 1902(a)(10)(A)(ii)(XVI) allows states to continue coverage for working individuals with disabilities whose medical conditions remain severe but who would otherwise lose SSI eligibility due to medical improvement as determined at a regularly scheduled continuing disability review. Eligibility is limited to individuals who cease to be eligible for the first TWWIIA buy-in due to medical improvement. States can impose premiums or other cost sharing based on income.

For both TWWIIA buy-ins, states may require premiums or cost sharing set on a sliding scale based on income. They may charge 100 percent of the premium to individuals whose income exceeds 250 percent FPL but is below 450 percent FPL, provided that these premiums do not exceed 7.5 percent of income. States must require payment of 100 percent of the premium for individuals whose adjusted gross income, as defined by the Internal Revenue Service, exceeds $75,000, except that a state may subsidize the premiums with

unmatched state funds. In order to receive federal matching funds for these buy-ins, states must meet a maintenance of effort requirement for funds that had previously been spent on state programs to enable people with disabilities to work, but this maintenance of effort requirement specifically excludes money spent for Medicaid.

Social Security Disability Insurance

The federal Social Security Disability Insurance (SSDI) program provides cash benefits to some individuals with a physical or mental impairment or blindness regardless of income level. In certain cases the disabled person's spouse or children can receive benefits as well. SSDI beneficiaries are generally eligible for Medicare two years after the onset of disability. Some individuals in this 24-month waiting period—and beyond, after they obtain Medicare coverage—have high medical expenses that lead them to "spend down" onto Medicaid, or low incomes that qualify them for Medicaid under another eligibility pathway. Individuals who are enrolled in both programs are referred to as dual eligibles.

Individuals qualify for SSDI based on their contributions to the Social Security Trust Fund through the Federal Insurance Contributions Act (FICA) Social Security tax paid on their earnings. In order to be eligible for SSDI an individual generally must have paid Social Security taxes for enough years to be covered under Social Security insurance; the number of years varies by the individual's age. The amount of monthly disability benefits is based on an individual's lifetime average earnings covered by Social Security.

The medical requirements for disability payments are the same under both SSDI and SSI, and the same process is used for both programs to determine disability. This includes not being able to work, or working but earning less than the SGA level.

The SSDI program also pays benefits to certain adults who have not worked enough to qualify for Social Security insurance (including some who have never worked). Their eligibility can be based on a parent's Social Security earnings record if they are currently or formerly dependent on that parent. These adults must be unmarried, and their disability must have begun before age 22. For disabled adults to become entitled to this benefit, one of their parents must be receiving Social Security retirement or disability benefits; or if deceased the parent must have worked long enough under Social Security to qualify for benefits. These benefits continue as long as the adult child remains disabled.

Methodology for Adjusting Benefit Spending Data

The FY 2008 Medicaid benefit spending amounts shown in the June 2011 MACStats were calculated based on Medicaid Statistical Information System (MSIS) data that have been adjusted to match total benefit spending reported by states in CMS-64 data.[45] Although the CMS-64 provides a more complete accounting of spending and is preferred when examining state or federal spending totals, MSIS is the only data source that allows for analysis of benefit spending by eligibility group and other enrollee characteristics.[46] We adjust the MSIS amounts for several reasons:

- CMS-64 data provide an official accounting of state spending on Medicaid for purposes of receiving federal matching dollars; in contrast, MSIS data are primarily used for statistical purposes.

- MSIS generally understates total Medicaid benefit spending because it excludes disproportionate share hospital (DSH) and additional types of supplemental payments made to hospitals and other providers, Medicare premium payments, and certain other amounts.[47]

- MSIS generally overstates net spending on prescribed drugs, because it excludes rebates from drug manufacturers.

- Even after accounting for differences in their scope and design, MSIS still tends to produce lower total benefit spending than the CMS-64.[48]

- The extent to which MSIS differs from the CMS-64 varies by state, meaning that a cross-state comparison of unadjusted MSIS amounts may not reflect true differences in benefit spending. See Table 13 for unadjusted benefit spending amounts in MSIS as a percentage of benefit spending in the CMS-64.

---

[45] Medicaid benefit spending reported here excludes the territories, administrative spending, the Vaccines for Children program (which is authorized by the Medicaid statute but operates as a separate program), and offsetting collections from third-party liability, estate, and other recoveries.

[46] For a discussion of these data sources, see MACPAC, Improving Medicaid and CHIP data for policy analysis and program accountability, in *Report to the Congress on Medicaid and CHIP: March 2011* (Washington, DC, MACPAC, 2011). http://www.macpac.gov/reports/MACPAC_March2011_web.pdf.

[47] Some of these amounts, including DSH and other supplemental payments, are lump sums not related to service use by an individual Medicaid enrollee. Nonetheless, we refer to these CMS-64 amounts as benefit spending, and the adjustment methodology described here distributes them across Medicaid enrollees with MSIS spending in the relevant service categories (e.g., hospital). We include both types of supplemental payments in benefit spending partly because unlike DSH, states do not reliably break out their non-DSH supplemental payments separately from their regular payments for hospital and other care in the CMS-64. If accurate reports of both DSH and non-DSH supplemental payments become available, we will consider an alternative adjustment methodology that excludes them.

[48] T. Plewes, *Databases for estimating health insurance coverage for children: A workshop summary* (Washington, DC: The National Academies Press, 2010):32-37. http://www.nap.edu/catalog/13024.html.

SECTION 4

MACStats

TABLE 13.   Medicaid Benefit Spending in MSIS and CMS-64 Data by State, FY 2008 (billions)

State	MSIS	CMS-64	MSIS as a Percentage of CMS-64
Total	$293.7	$338.6	86.7%
Alabama	3.5	4.1	86.0
Alaska	0.9	0.9	106.4
Arizona	6.6	7.5	87.7
Arkansas	3.2	3.3	96.1
California	32.0	39.0	82.1
Colorado	3.0	3.2	94.2
Connecticut	4.1	4.5	91.2
Delaware	1.1	1.1	103.2
District of Columbia	1.7	1.4	119.4
Florida	13.2	14.7	90.0
Georgia	6.9	7.3	93.5
Hawaii	1.0	1.2	80.3
Idaho	1.2	1.2	102.8
Illinois	10.1	11.6	87.3
Indiana	4.9	6.2	78.9
Iowa	2.7	2.8	94.3
Kansas	2.3	2.3	100.9
Kentucky	4.4	4.8	91.2
Louisiana	4.8	6.1	79.2
Maine	1.4	2.3	60.0
Maryland	5.4	5.7	94.0
Massachusetts	8.8	10.8	81.0
Michigan	9.2	9.8	93.5
Minnesota	6.6	7.0	95.2
Mississippi	3.1	3.8	81.9
Missouri	5.1	7.1	71.8
Montana	0.7	0.8	84.3
Nebraska	1.5	1.6	92.9
Nevada	1.1	1.3	85.8
New Hampshire	0.9	1.3	74.4
New Jersey	7.4	9.4	78.3
New Mexico	2.9	3.0	95.7
New York	43.0	47.6	90.4
North Carolina	8.8	10.2	87.0
North Dakota	0.5	0.5	101.9
Ohio	11.6	12.4	93.2
Oklahoma	3.2	3.5	90.8
Oregon	2.5	3.2	76.4
Pennsylvania	12.5	16.3	76.7
Rhode Island	1.6	1.8	85.6
South Carolina	4.3	4.4	96.1
South Dakota	0.7	0.7	99.9
Tennessee	6.3	7.2	87.8
Texas	16.7	21.5	77.6
Utah	1.6	1.5	108.3
Vermont	0.9	1.1	81.7
Virginia	4.6	5.4	86.1
Washington	5.8	6.3	92.7
West Virginia	2.4	2.3	105.5
Wisconsin	4.5	5.0	89.3
Wyoming	0.5	0.5	102.1

Note: See text for a discussion of differences between MSIS and CMS-64 data. Both sources are unadjusted. The CMS-64 amounts exclude $5.5 billion in offsetting collections from third-party liability, estate, and other recoveries.

Source: MACPAC analysis of MSIS Annual Person Summary (APS) data and CMS-64 Financial Management Report (FMR) net expenditure data from CMS

SECTION 4

MACStats

The methodology MACPAC uses for adjusting the MSIS benefit spending data involves the following steps:

» We aggregate the service types into broad categories that are comparable between the two sources. This is necessary because there is not a one-to-one correspondence of service types in the MSIS and CMS-64 data. Even service types that have identical names may still be reported differently in the two sources due to differences in the instructions given to states. Table 14 provides additional detail on the categories used.

» We calculate state-specific adjustment factors for each of the service categories by dividing CMS-64 benefit spending by MSIS benefit spending.

» We then multiply MSIS dollar amounts in each service category by the state-specific factors to obtain adjusted MSIS spending. For example, in a state with a fee-for-service hospital factor of 1.2, each Medicaid enrollee with hospital spending in MSIS would have that spending multiplied by 1.2; doing so makes the sum of adjusted hospital spending amounts among individual Medicaid enrollees in MSIS total the aggregate hospital spending reported by states in the CMS-64.[49]

By making these adjustments to the MSIS data, we are attempting to provide comparable estimates of Medicaid benefit spending across states that can be analyzed by eligibility group and other enrollee characteristics. There are a number of areas where this methodology might be refined

for future analyses—for example, with regard to the services included in the long-term services and supports category and the treatment of DSH and other supplemental payments that are not related to service use by an individual Medicaid enrollee. Other organizations, including the Office of the Actuary at CMS, the Kaiser Commission on Medicaid and the Uninsured, and the Urban Institute, use methodologies that are similar to MACPAC's but may differ in various ways—for example, by using different service categories or producing estimates for future years based on actual data for earlier years.

Managed Care Enrollment and Spending Guide

There are four main sources of data on Medicaid managed care available from CMS.

The Medicaid Managed Care Data Collection System (MMCDCS) provides aggregate enrollment statistics and other basic information for each managed care plan within a state. CMS uses the MMCDCS to create an annual *Medicaid Managed Care Enrollment Report*,[50] which is the source of information on Medicaid managed care most commonly cited by CMS, as well as outside analysts and researchers. CMS also uses the MMCDCS to produce an annual *National Summary of State Medicaid Managed Care Programs* that describes the managed care programs within a state (generally defined by the statutory authority under which they operate),[51] each of which may include several managed care plans.

---

[49] The sum of adjusted MSIS benefit spending amounts for all service categories totals CMS-64 benefit spending, exclusive of offsetting collections from third-party liability, estate, and other recoveries. These collections, $5.5 billion in FY 2008, are not reported by type of service in the CMS-64 and are not reported at all in MSIS.

[50] CMS, *Medicaid managed care enrollment report*, https://www.cms.gov/MedicaidDataSourcesGenInfo/04_MdManCrEnrllRep.asp.

[51] CMS, *Description of state programs*, https://www.cms.gov/MedicaidDataSourcesGenInfo/06_DescStateProg.asp.

SECTION 4

MACStats

TABLE 14. Service Categories Used to Adjust Medicaid Benefit Spending in MSIS to Match CMS-64 Totals

Service Category	MSIS Service Types	CMS-64 Service Types
Hospital	▷ Inpatient hospital ▷ Outpatient hospital ▷ Inpatient psychiatric for under age 21 ▷ Mental health facility for the aged	▷ Inpatient hospital regular payments ▷ Inpatient hospital non-DSH supplemental payments ▷ Inpatient hospital DSH ▷ Mental health facility regular payments ▷ Mental health facility DSH ▷ Outpatient hospital regular payments ▷ Outpatient hospital supplemental payments ▷ Critical access hospital ▷ Emergency hospital ▷ Emergency services for aliens[1]
Non-hospital acute care	▷ Physician ▷ Dental ▷ Nurse midwife ▷ Nurse practitioner ▷ Other practitioner ▷ Non-hospital outpatient clinic ▷ Lab/X-ray ▷ Sterilizations ▷ Abortions ▷ Physical, occupational, speech, and hearing therapy	▷ Physician regular payments ▷ Physician supplemental payments ▷ Dental ▷ Nurse midwife ▷ Nurse practitioner ▷ Other practitioner regular payments ▷ Other practitioner supplemental payments ▷ Non-hospital outpatient clinic ▷ Rural health clinic ▷ Federally qualified health center ▷ Lab/X-ray ▷ Sterilizations ▷ Abortions ▷ EPSDT screenings ▷ Non-emergency transportation ▷ Physical, occupational, speech, and hearing therapy ▷ Prosthetics, dentures, and eyeglasses ▷ Diagnostic screening and preventive services ▷ School-based services ▷ Care not otherwise categorized
Drugs	▷ Drugs (gross spending)	▷ Drugs (gross spending) ▷ Drug rebates

TABLE 14, Continued

Service Category	MSIS Service Types	CMS-64 Service Types
Managed care and premium assistance	‣ HMO (i.e., comprehensive risk-based managed care; includes PACE) ‣ PHP ‣ PCCM	‣ MCO (i.e., comprehensive risk-based managed care) ‣ PAHP ‣ PIHP ‣ PCCM ‣ PACE ‣ Premium assistance for employer-sponsored coverage
LTSS non-institutional	‣ Home health ‣ Personal care ‣ Private duty nursing ‣ Targeted case management ‣ Rehabilitative services ‣ Hospice ‣ Other services (consists primarily of HCB waiver)	‣ Home health ‣ Personal care ‣ Private duty nursing ‣ Case management (excludes primary care case management) ‣ Rehabilitative services ‣ Hospice ‣ HCB waiver and state plan services
LTSS institutional	‣ Nursing facility ‣ ICF/MR	‣ Nursing facility regular payments ‣ Nursing facility supplemental payments ‣ ICF/MR regular payments ‣ ICF/MR supplemental payments
Medicare[2,3]		‣ Medicare Part A and Part B premiums ‣ Medicare coinsurance and deductibles for QMBs

Notes: EPSDT = Early and Periodic Screening, Diagnostic, and Treatment; HCB = home and community-based; HMO = health maintenance organization; ICF/MR = intermediate care facility for the mentally retarded; LTSS = long-term services and supports; MCO = managed care organization; PACE = Program of All-Inclusive Care for the Elderly; PHP = prepaid health plan, either a PAHP or a PIHP; PAHP = prepaid ambulatory health plan; PIHP = prepaid inpatient health plan; PCCM = primary care case management; QMB = Qualified Medicare Beneficiary.

Service categories and types reflect fee-for-service spending unless noted otherwise. Service types with identical names in the MSIS and CMS-64 may still be reported differently in the two sources due to differences in the instructions given to states; amounts for those that appear only in the CMS-64 (e.g., DSH) are distributed across Medicaid enrollees with MSIS spending in the relevant service categories (e.g., hospital).

1 Emergency services for aliens are reported under individual service types throughout MSIS, but primarily inpatient and outpatient hospital. As a result, we include this CMS-64 amount in the hospital category.

2 Medicare premiums are not reported in MSIS. We distribute CMS-64 amounts across dual eligible enrollees in MSIS.

3 Medicare coinsurance and deductibles are reported under individual service types throughout MSIS. We distribute the CMS-64 amount for QMBs across CMS-64 spending in the hospital and non-hospital acute categories prior to calculating adjustment factors, based on the distribution of spending for these categories among QMBs in MSIS.

Source: MACPAC analysis of MSIS and CMS-64 data

SECTION 4

MACStats

The Medicaid Statistical Information System (MSIS) provides person-level and claims-level information for all Medicaid enrollees.[52] With regard to managed care, the information collected for each enrollee includes plan ID numbers and types for up to four managed care plans (including comprehensive risk-based plans, PCCMs, and limited-benefit plans) under which the enrollee is covered; if enrolled in a 1915(b) or other waiver, the waiver ID number; claims that provide a record of each capitated payment made on behalf of the enrollee to a managed care plan (these are generally referred to as capitated claims); and, in some states, a record of each service received by the enrollee from a provider under contract with a managed care plan (these generally do not include a payment amount and are referred to as encounter or "dummy" claims). As discussed in the managed care sections of this Report and in MACPAC's March 2011 Report to the Congress, all states collect encounter data from their Medicaid managed care plans, but some do not report it in MSIS. Managed care enrollees may also have FFS claims in MSIS if they used services that were not included in their managed care plan's contract with the state.

The CMS-64 provides aggregate spending information for Medicaid by major benefit categories, including managed care. The spending amounts reported by states on the CMS-64 are used to calculate their federal matching dollars.

The Statistical Enrollment Data System (SEDS) provides aggregate statistics on CHIP enrollment and child Medicaid enrollment that include the number covered under fee for service and managed care systems. SEDS is the only comprehensive source of information on managed care participation among separate CHIP enrollees

across states; however, it is generally not used to examine managed care participation among Medicaid-expansion CHIP and regular Medicaid enrollees, for which other data sources are available.

In MACStats and the managed care chapter of this Report, many of the statistics cited on managed care are from CMS's *2009 Medicaid Managed Care Enrollment Report*. However, the enrollment report does not provide information on characteristics of enrollees in managed care aside from dual eligibility status (e.g., basis of eligibility and demographics such as age, sex, and race/ethnicity) or their spending and non-managed care service use. As a result, we supplement statistics from the enrollment report with MSIS and CMS-64 data; for example, Tables 11 and 12 use MSIS data to show the percentage of child, adult, disabled, and aged Medicaid enrollees who are enrolled in managed care and the percentage of their Medicaid benefit spending that was for managed care.

When examining managed care statistics from various sources, the following issues should be noted:

▸ Figures in the annual Medicaid Managed Care Enrollment Report published by CMS include Medicaid-expansion CHIP enrollees. Although we generally exclude these children (about 2 million, depending on the time period) from Medicaid analyses, it is not possible to do so with the enrollment report data cited for Tables 9 and 10 in MACStats and throughout the managed care chapter. Tables 11 and 12—which show the percentage of child, adult, disabled, and aged Medicaid enrollees who are enrolled in managed care and the percentage of their Medicaid benefit spending that was for

---

[52] For enrollees with no paid claims during a given period (e.g., fiscal year), their MSIS data are limited to person-level information (e.g., basis of eligibility, age, sex, etc.).

managed care—are based on MSIS data and exclude Medicaid-expansion CHIP enrollees.[53]

> The types of managed care reported by states may differ somewhat between the Medicaid Managed Care Enrollment Report and the MSIS. For example, in their MSIS data, Alabama, Idaho, and Utah report a small number of enrollees in comprehensive risk-based managed care (Table 11); in their enrollment report data, they report zero enrollees in this category (Table 9). Anomalies in the MSIS data are documented by CMS as it reviews each state's quarterly submission,[54] but not all issues may be identified in this process.

> The Medicaid Managed Care enrollment report provides point-in-time figures (e.g., as of June 30, 2009). In contrast, CMS generally uses MSIS to report on the number of enrollees ever in managed care during a fiscal year (although point-in-time enrollment can also be calculated from MSIS based on the monthly data it contains).

SECTION 4

MACStats

---

[53] We generally exclude Medicaid-expansion children from Medicaid analyses because their funding stream (CHIP, under Title XXI of the Social Security Act) differs from that of other Medicaid enrollees (Medicaid, under Title XIX). In addition, spending (and often enrollment) for the Medicaid-expansion CHIP population is reported by CMS in CHIP statistics, along with information on separate CHIP enrollees.

[54] See CMS, MSIS *State Anomalies/Issues*, 2009. http://www.cms.gov/MedicaidDataSourcesGenInfo/02_MSISData.asp.

Acronym List

AAA	American Academy of Actuaries
ACG	Adjusted Clinical Group
ACO	Accountable Care Organization
ADL	Activity of Daily Living
AFDC	Aid to Families with Dependent Children
ASO	Administrative Service Organization
ASOP	Actuarial Standard of Practice
BBA	Balanced Budget Act
CAHPS	Consumer Assessment of Healthcare Providers and Systems
CBO	Congressional Budget Office
CDPS	Chronic Illness and Disability Payment System
CHC	Community Health Center
CHIP	State Children's Health Insurance Program
CHIPRA	Children's Health Insurance Program Reauthorization Act of 2009
CMS	Centers for Medicare & Medicaid Services
CRxG	Clinical Risk Group – Pharmacy Add-on
CSHCN	Children With Special Health Care Needs
DRA	Deficit Reduction Act
DRG	Diagnosis Related Group
DSH	Disproportionate Share Hospital
D-SNP	Dual Eligible Special Needs Plan
DxCG	Medicaid Rx Diagnostic Cost Group
ED	Emergency Department
E-FMAP	Enhanced Federal Medical Assistance Percentage
EPSDT	Early and Periodic Screening, Diagnostic and Treatment
EQR	External Quality Review
EQRO	External Quality Review Organization
EWS	Early-Warning System
FCHCO	Federal Coordinated Health Care Office
FFS	Fee for Service
FMAP	Federal Medical Assistance Percentage

FPL	Federal Poverty Level
FQHC	Federally Qualified Health Center
FUL	Federal Upper Limit
FY	Fiscal Year
GAO	Government Accountability Office
GDP	Gross Domestic Product
HCBS	Home and Community-Based Services
HCFA	Health Care Financing Administration (now CMS)
HEDIS	Healthcare Effectiveness Data and Information Set
HHS	United States Department of Health and Human Services
HIO	Health Insuring Organization
HMO	Health Maintenance Organization
HMOA	Health Maintenance Organization Act
HPSA	Health Professional Shortage Area
HRSA	Health Resource and Services Administration
ICF/MR	Intermediate Care Facilities for the Mentally Retarded
IOM	Institute of Medicine
LTC	Long-Term Care
LTSS	Long-Term Support and Services
MA	Medicare Advantage
MACPAC	Medicaid and CHIP Payment and Access Commission
MAGI	Modified Adjusted Gross Income
MAX	Medicaid Analytic eXtract
MCE	Managed Care Entity
MCH	Maternal and Child Health
MCO	Managed Care Organization
MedPAC	Medicare Payment Advisory Commission
MFCU	Medicaid Fraud Control Unit
MIP	Medicaid Integrity Program
MIPPA	Medicare Improvements for Patients and Providers Act
MMCDCS	Medicaid Managed Care Data Collection System
MMIS	Medicaid Management Information System
MOE	Maintenance of Effort
MSIS	Medicaid Statistical Information System
NAMD	National Association of Medicaid Directors
NCQA	National Committee for Quality Assurance

NF	Nursing Facility
OACT	CMS Office of the Actuary
OBRA	Omnibus Reconciliation Act
OIG	Office of the Inspector General
PACE	Program of All Inclusive Care for the Elderly
PAHP	Prepaid Ambulatory Health Plan
PCP	Primary Care Provider
PI	Program Integrity
PIHP	Prepaid Inpatient Health Plan
PPACA	Patient Protection and Affordable Care Act
PCCM	Primary Care Case Management
POS	Point-of-Service
PMPM	Per Member Per Month
PPO	Preferred Provider Organization
RFP	Request for Proposal
RHC	Rural Health Clinic
SEDS	Statistical Enrollment Data System
SFY	State Fiscal Year
SNP	Special Needs Plan
SPA	State Plan Amendment
SSA	Social Security Act
SSI	Supplemental Security Income
TANF	Temporary Assistance for Needy Families
UPL	Upper Payment Limit

Authorizing Language from the Social Security Act (42 U.S.C. 1396)

MEDICAID AND CHIP PAYMENT AND ACCESS COMMISSION

(a) ESTABLISHMENT.—There is hereby established the Medicaid and CHIP Payment and Access Commission (in this section referred to as 'MACPAC').

(b) DUTIES.—

(1) REVIEW OF ACCESS POLICIES FOR ALL STATES AND ANNUAL REPORTS.—MACPAC shall—

(A) review policies of the Medicaid program established under this title (in this section referred to as 'Medicaid') and the State Children's Health Insurance Program established under title XXI (in this section referred to as 'CHIP') affecting access to covered items and services, including topics described in paragraph (2);

(B) make recommendations to Congress, the Secretary, and States concerning such access policies;

(C) by not later than March 15 of each year (beginning with 2010), submit a report to Congress containing the results of such reviews and MACPAC's recommendations concerning such policies; and

(D) by not later than June 15 of each year (beginning with 2010), submit a report to Congress containing an examination of issues affecting Medicaid and CHIP, including the implications of changes in health care delivery in the United States and in the market for health care services on such programs.

(2) SPECIFIC TOPICS TO BE REVIEWED.—Specifically, MACPAC shall review and assess the following:

(A) MEDICAID AND CHIP PAYMENT POLICIES.—Payment policies under Medicaid and CHIP, including—

(i) the factors affecting expenditures for the efficient provision of items and services in different sectors, including the process for updating payments to medical, dental, and health professionals, hospitals, residential and long-term care providers, providers of home and community based services, Federally-qualified health centers and rural health clinics, managed care entities, and providers of other covered items and services;

(ii) payment methodologies; and

(iii) the relationship of such factors and methodologies to access and quality of care for Medicaid and CHIP beneficiaries (including how such factors and methodologies enable such beneficiaries to obtain the services for which they are eligible, affect provider supply, and affect providers that serve a disproportionate share of low-income and other vulnerable populations).

(B) ELIGIBILITY POLICIES.—Medicaid and CHIP eligibility policies, including a determination of the degree to which Federal and State policies provide health care coverage to needy populations.

(C) ENROLLMENT AND RETENTION PROCESSES.—Medicaid and CHIP enrollment and retention processes, including a determination of the degree to which Federal and State policies encourage the enrollment of individuals who are eligible for such programs and screen out individuals who are ineligible, while minimizing the share of program expenses devoted to such processes.

(D) COVERAGE POLICIES.—Medicaid and CHIP benefit and coverage policies, including a determination of the degree to which Federal and State policies provide access to the services enrollees require to improve and maintain their health and functional status.

(E) QUALITY OF CARE.—Medicaid and CHIP policies as they relate to the quality of care provided under those programs, including a determination of the degree to which Federal and State policies achieve their stated goals and interact with similar goals established by other purchasers of health care services.

(F) INTERACTION OF MEDICAID AND CHIP PAYMENT POLICIES WITH HEALTH CARE DELIVERY GENERALLY.—The effect of Medicaid and CHIP payment policies on access to items and services for children and other Medicaid and CHIP populations other than under this title or title XXI and the implications of changes in health care delivery in the United States and in the general market for health care items and services on Medicaid and CHIP.

(G) INTERACTIONS WITH MEDICARE AND MEDICAID.— Consistent with paragraph (11), the interaction of policies under Medicaid and the Medicare program under title XVIII, including with respect to how such interactions affect access to services, payments, and dual eligible individuals.

(H) OTHER ACCESS POLICIES.—The effect of other Medicaid and CHIP policies on access to covered items and services, including policies relating to transportation and language barriers and preventive, acute, and long-term services and supports.

(3) RECOMMENDATIONS AND REPORTS OF STATE-SPECIFIC DATA.—MACPAC shall—

(A) review national and State-specific Medicaid and CHIP data; and

(B) submit reports and recommendations to Congress, the Secretary, and States based on such reviews.

(4) CREATION OF EARLY-WARNING SYSTEM.—MACPAC shall create an early-warning system to identify provider shortage areas, as well as other factors that adversely affect, or have the potential to adversely affect, access to care by, or the health care status of, Medicaid and CHIP beneficiaries. MACPAC shall include in the annual report required under paragraph (1)(D) a description of all such areas or problems identified with respect to the period addressed in the report.

(5) COMMENTS ON CERTAIN SECRETARIAL REPORTS AND REGULATIONS.—

   (A) CERTAIN SECRETARIAL REPORTS.—If the Secretary submits to Congress (or a committee of Congress) a report that is required by law and that relates to access policies, including with respect to payment policies, under Medicaid or CHIP, the Secretary shall transmit a copy of the report to MACPAC. MACPAC shall review the report and, not later than 6 months after the date of submittal of the Secretary's report to Congress, shall submit to the appropriate committees of Congress and the Secretary written comments on such report. Such comments may include such recommendations as MACPAC deems appropriate.

   (B) REGULATIONS.—MACPAC shall review Medicaid and CHIP regulations and may comment through submission of a report to the appropriate committees of Congress and the Secretary, on any such regulations that affect access, quality, or efficiency of health care.

(6) AGENDA AND ADDITIONAL REVIEWS.—MACPAC shall consult periodically with the chairmen and ranking minority members of the appropriate committees of Congress regarding MACPAC's agenda and progress towards achieving the agenda. MACPAC may conduct additional reviews, and submit additional reports to the appropriate committees of Congress, from time to time on such topics relating to the program under this title or title XXI as may be requested by such chairmen and members and as MACPAC deems appropriate.

(7) AVAILABILITY OF REPORTS.—MACPAC shall transmit to the Secretary a copy of each report submitted under this subsection and shall make such reports available to the public.

(8) APPROPRIATE COMMITTEE OF CONGRESS.—For purposes of this section, the term 'appropriate committees of Congress' means the Committee on Energy and Commerce of the House of Representatives and the Committee on Finance of the Senate.

(9) VOTING AND REPORTING REQUIREMENTS.—With respect to each recommendation contained in a report submitted under paragraph (1), each member of MACPAC shall vote on the recommendation, and MACPAC shall include, by member, the results of that vote in the report containing the recommendation.

(10) EXAMINATION OF BUDGET CONSEQUENCES.—Before making any recommendations, MACPAC shall examine the budget consequences of such recommendations, directly or through consultation with appropriate expert entities, and shall submit with any recommendations, a report on the Federal and State-specific budget consequences of the recommendations.

(11) CONSULTATION AND COORDINATION WITH MEDPAC.—

   (A) IN GENERAL.—MACPAC shall consult with the Medicare Payment Advisory Commission (in this paragraph referred to as 'MedPAC') established under section 1805 in carrying out its duties under this section, as appropriate and particularly with respect to the issues specified in paragraph (2) as they relate to those Medicaid beneficiaries who are dually eligible for Medicaid and the Medicare program under title XVIII, adult Medicaid beneficiaries (who are not dually eligible for Medicare), and beneficiaries under Medicare. Responsibility for analysis of and recommendations to change Medicare policy regarding Medicare beneficiaries, including Medicare beneficiaries who are dually eligible for Medicare and Medicaid, shall rest with MedPAC.

   (B) INFORMATION SHARING.—MACPAC and MedPAC shall have access to deliberations and records of the other such entity, respectively, upon the request of the other such entity.

(12) CONSULTATION WITH STATES.—MACPAC shall regularly consult with States in carrying out its duties under this section, including with respect to developing processes for carrying out such duties, and shall ensure that input from States is taken into account and represented in MACPAC's recommendations and reports.

(13) COORDINATE AND CONSULT WITH THE FEDERAL COORDINATED HEALTH CARE OFFICE.—MACPAC shall coordinate and consult with the Federal Coordinated Health Care Office established under section 2081 of the Patient Protection and Affordable Care Act before making any recommendations regarding dual eligible individuals.

(14) PROGRAMMATIC OVERSIGHT VESTED IN THE SECRETARY.—MACPAC's authority to make recommendations in accordance with this section shall not affect, or be considered to duplicate, the Secretary's authority to carry out Federal responsibilities with respect to Medicaid and CHIP.

(c) MEMBERSHIP.—

(1) NUMBER AND APPOINTMENT.—MACPAC shall be composed of 17 members appointed by the Comptroller General of the United States.

(2) QUALIFICATIONS.—

(A) IN GENERAL.—The membership of MACPAC shall include individuals who have had direct experience as enrollees or parents or caregivers of enrollees in Medicaid or CHIP and individuals with national recognition for their expertise in Federal safety net health programs, health finance and economics, actuarial science, health plans and integrated delivery systems, reimbursement for health care, health information technology, and other providers of health services, public health, and other related fields, who provide a mix of different professions, broad geographic representation, and a balance between urban and rural representation.

(B) INCLUSION.—The membership of MACPAC shall include (but not be limited to) physicians, dentists, and other health professionals, employers, third-party payers, and individuals with expertise in the delivery of health services. Such membership shall also include representatives of children, pregnant women, the elderly, individuals with disabilities, caregivers, and dual eligible individuals, current or former representatives of State agencies responsible for administering Medicaid, and current or former representatives of State agencies responsible for administering CHIP.

(C) MAJORITY NONPROVIDERS.—Individuals who are directly involved in the provision, or management of the delivery, of items and services covered under Medicaid or CHIP shall not constitute a majority of the membership of MACPAC.

(D) ETHICAL DISCLOSURE.—The Comptroller General of the United States shall establish a system for public disclosure by members of MACPAC of financial and other potential conflicts of interest relating to such members. Members of MACPAC shall be treated as employees of Congress for purposes of applying title I of the Ethics in Government Act of 1978 (Public Law 95–521).

(3) TERMS.—

(A) IN GENERAL.—The terms of members of MACPAC shall be for 3 years except that the Comptroller General of the United States shall designate staggered terms for the members first appointed.

(B) VACANCIES.—Any member appointed to fill a vacancy occurring before the expiration of the term for which the member's predecessor was appointed shall be appointed only for the remainder of that term. A member may serve after the expiration of that member's term until a successor has taken office. A vacancy in MACPAC shall be filled in the manner in which the original appointment was made.

(4) COMPENSATION.—While serving on the business of MACPAC (including travel time), a member of MACPAC shall be entitled to compensation at the per diem equivalent of the rate provided for level IV of the Executive Schedule under section 5315 of title 5, United States Code; and while so serving away from home and the member's regular place of business, a member may be allowed travel expenses, as authorized by the Chairman of MACPAC. Physicians serving as personnel of MACPAC may be provided a physician comparability allowance by MACPAC in the same manner as Government physicians may be provided such an allowance by an agency under section 5948 of title 5, United States Code, and for such purpose subsection (i) of such section shall apply to MACPAC in the same manner as it applies to the Tennessee Valley Authority. For purposes of pay (other than pay of members of MACPAC) and employment benefits, rights, and privileges, all personnel of MACPAC shall be treated as if they were employees of the United States Senate.

(5) CHAIRMAN; VICE CHAIRMAN.—The Comptroller General of the United States shall designate a member of MACPAC, at the time of appointment of the member as Chairman and a member as Vice Chairman for that term of appointment, except that in the case of vacancy of the Chairmanship or Vice Chairmanship, the Comptroller General of the United States may designate another member for the remainder of that member's term.

(6) MEETINGS.—MACPAC shall meet at the call of the Chairman.

(d) DIRECTOR AND STAFF; EXPERTS AND CONSULTANTS.—Subject to such review as the Comptroller General of the United States deems necessary to assure the efficient administration of MACPAC, MACPAC may—

(1) employ and fix the compensation of an Executive Director (subject to the approval of the Comptroller General of the United States) and such other personnel as may be necessary to carry out its duties (without regard to the provisions of title 5, United States Code, governing appointments in the competitive service);

(2) seek such assistance and support as may be required in the performance of its duties from appropriate Federal and State departments and agencies;

(3) enter into contracts or make other arrangements, as may be necessary for the conduct of the work of MACPAC (without regard to section 3709 of the Revised Statutes (41 U.S.C. 5));

(4) make advance, progress, and other payments which relate to the work of MACPAC;

(5) provide transportation and subsistence for persons serving without compensation; and

(6) prescribe such rules and regulations as it deems necessary with respect to the internal organization and operation of MACPAC.

(e) POWERS.—

    (1) OBTAINING OFFICIAL DATA.—MACPAC may secure directly from any department or agency of the United States and, as a condition for receiving payments under sections 1903(a) and 2105(a), from any State agency responsible for administering Medicaid or CHIP, information necessary to enable it to carry out this section. Upon request of the Chairman, the head of that department or agency shall furnish that information to MACPAC on an agreed upon schedule.

    (2) DATA COLLECTION.—In order to carry out its functions, MACPAC shall—

        (A) utilize existing information, both published and unpublished, where possible, collected and assessed either by its own staff or under other arrangements made in accordance with this section;

        (B) carry out, or award grants or contracts for, original research and experimentation, where existing information is inadequate; and

        (C) adopt procedures allowing any interested party to submit information for MACPAC's use in making reports and recommendations.

    (3) ACCESS OF GAO TO INFORMATION.—The Comptroller General of the United States shall have unrestricted access to all deliberations, records, and nonproprietary data of MACPAC, immediately upon request.

    (4) PERIODIC AUDIT.—MACPAC shall be subject to periodic audit by the Comptroller General of the United States.

(f) FUNDING.—

    (1) REQUEST FOR APPROPRIATIONS.—MACPAC shall submit requests for appropriations (other than for fiscal year 2010) in the same manner as the Comptroller General of the United States submits requests for appropriations, but amounts appropriated for MACPAC shall be separate from amounts appropriated for the Comptroller General of the United States.

    (2) AUTHORIZATION.—There are authorized to be appropriated such sums as may be necessary to carry out the provisions of this section.

    (3) FUNDING FOR FISCAL YEAR 2010.—

        (A) IN GENERAL.—Out of any funds in the Treasury not otherwise appropriated, there is appropriated to MACPAC to carry out the provisions of this section for fiscal year 2010, $9,000,000.

        (B) TRANSFER OF FUNDS.—Notwithstanding section 2104(a)(13), from the amounts appropriated in such section for fiscal year 2010, $2,000,000 is hereby transferred and made available in such fiscal year to MACPAC to carry out the provisions of this section.

    (4) AVAILABILITY.—Amounts made available under paragraphs (2) and (3) to MACPAC to carry out the provisions of this section shall remain available until expended.

Additional MACPAC Requirements— Excerpt from Sec. 399V-4 of 42 U.S.C. 280g-15

State Demonstration Programs to Evaluate Alternatives to Current Medical Tort Litigation

The Patient Protection and Accountable Care Act also amended the Public Health Service Act (PHSA) to require MACPAC to "conduct an independent review of the alternatives to current tort litigation that are implemented under grants under subsection (a) [of Sec. 399V-4 of the PHSA, entitled 'State Demonstration Programs to Evaluate Alternatives to Current Medical Tort Litigation'] to determine the impact of such alternatives on the Medicaid or CHIP programs … and their beneficiaries." Subsection (h) requires that, "[n]ot later than December 31, 2016, the Medicare Payment Advisory Commission [MedPAC] and the Medicaid and CHIP Payment and Access Commission [MACPAC] shall each submit to Congress a report that includes the findings and recommendations of each respective Commission based on [their] independent reviews … , including an analysis of the impact of the alternatives reviewed on the efficiency and effectiveness of the respective programs."

Commission's Deliberations on Managed Care in Medicaid

October 2010—May 2011

The Commission established Medicaid managed care as a key policy priority in its earliest deliberations. Since October 2010, the Commission has included Medicaid managed care issues in most of its public meetings. The Commission heard from states and plans and plan representatives on the issues facing them today and in the future. In addition, the Commission convened an Expert Roundtable comprised of leading state officials, researchers and health care industry representatives to discuss challenges and opportunities facing Medicaid managed care.

Based on expert presentations and public comments during the public meetings, the Commissioners examined key policy questions related to Medicaid managed care programs, reviewed policy issues, identified informational needs, and developed analytic work plans for future in-depth work on managed care issues in Medicaid.

Public Meetings	Summary of Commission's Discussion
October 28–29, 2010	Reviewed introductory information about Medicaid managed care, including: • A brief history of Medicaid managed care • National and state enrollment trends • Types of managed care models • Unique issues in Medicaid managed care design Developed a preliminary research agenda to guide work on Medicaid managed care for the June 2011 Report to the Congress
December 9–10, 2010	Examined findings from a literature review on Medicaid managed care Reviewed a summary of the discussion from an Expert Roundtable on Medicaid Managed care in October 2010 Key discussion topics included: • Impact of state budget conditions on Medicaid managed care policies • Provider network adequacy requirements and access to care, including oral health services • Payment methodologies and risk adjustment • Use of encounter data at the federal and state level • Federal and state monitoring and oversight Identified and provided guidance on critical policies and required analyses for future work on Medicaid managed care

Public Meetings	Summary of Commission's Discussion
April 14, 2011	▷ Representatives of Medicaid managed care plans testified before the Commission about plans' current and future priorities and challenges, including: ▪ Payment issues ▪ State enrollment and eligibility policies ▪ Enrolling high-cost, high-need populations into managed care ▷ Reviewed preliminary results from a MACPAC questionnaire that asked states to describe how they monitor and identify potential problems with access to care and provider capacity in their Medicaid managed care and fee-for-service programs ▷ Provided guidance for staff work for examining different managed care models
May 19, 2011	▷ State Medicaid Directors testified before the Commission to discuss: ▪ Differences between and experiences with comprehensive risk-based managed care and Primary Care Case Management (PCCM) programs ▪ The state's rationale for pursuing this delivery model, and ▪ Key concerns today as well as the opportunities and challenges facing them in the future in enrolling high-cost, high-need populations and addressing ways to promote efficiency and economy in state Medicaid programs ▷ Discussed and approved the content of Medicaid and CHIP managed care information that is presented in the June 2011 Report to the Congress

For additional information on the Commission's public meetings, go to http://www.macpac.gov/home/meetings to access meeting agendas, transcripts and presentations.

Consultations with States and Other Stakeholders

The Commission is statutorily charged to collaborate and consult with the congressional committees that have jurisdiction for MACPAC, as well as states, the Medicare Payment Advisory Commission (MedPAC), and the Federal Coordinated Health Care Office (FCHCO). MACPAC staff maintains active communication with these groups and with several other stakeholders to discuss Medicaid and CHIP-related activities and priorities.

Statutorily Required Consultation Activities

Congressional Committees of Jurisdiction: *(b)(6) AGENDA AND ADDITIONAL REVIEWS.—*
MACPAC shall consult periodically with the chairmen and ranking minority members of the appropriate committees of Congress regarding MACPAC's agenda and progress towards achieving the agenda. MACPAC may conduct additional reviews, and submit additional reports to the appropriate committees of Congress, from time to time on such topics relating to the program under this title or title XXI as may be requested by such chairmen and members and as MACPAC deems appropriate.

The Commission actively consults with the Senate Finance and House Energy and Commerce Committees, which have jurisdiction over Medicaid and CHIP. On an ongoing basis the Commission collaborates with key staff of these congressional committees, discussing priorities for our analytic work and receiving their input on issues discussed in public meetings. Prior to each public Commission meeting, the Commission briefs the staff, reviews the upcoming agenda and collects feedback on meeting sessions and analytic work plans. Additionally, congressional staff members have addressed the Commission to outline congressional priorities for the Medicaid and CHIP programs. Lastly, Commission staff provides technical assistance to congressional staff on various policy issues.

State Policy Officials and State-related Associations: *(b)(12) CONSULTATION WITH STATES.—*
MACPAC shall regularly consult with States in carrying out its duties under this section, including with respect to developing processes for carrying out such duties, and shall ensure that input from States is taken into account and represented in MACPAC's recommendations and reports.

The joint federal-state structure of Medicaid and CHIP requires that state perspectives and insight on emerging trends and policy issues be taken into account as the Commission develops independent policy analysis for the Congress. The Commission meets regularly with state Medicaid officials and other state-based associations to better understand state Medicaid data, programmatic information, and perspectives on emerging trends in the Medicaid and CHIP programs. To that end, the Commission has sought opportunities to collect targeted state data and information and incorporate state perspectives in

Commission meeting discussions. Almost every public Commission meeting has featured presentations by current or former state Medicaid and/or CHIP policy officials, during which state representatives add to the Commissioners' discussion on agenda topics and provide examples of how they have addressed payment, access, data, and other Medicaid and CHIP programmatic issues in their states. Prior to each public meeting, the Commission reviews the agenda with the National Association of Medicaid Directors (NAMD), the National Conference of State Legislatures (NCSL), the National Governors Association (NGA), the Southern Governors Association (SGA), the National Association of State Budget Officers (NASBO), and the National Academy of State Health Policy (NASHP).

To improve our understanding of states' perspectives in Commission analyses, staff are working with the NAMD and the Robert Wood Johnson Medicaid Leadership Institute Fellows (comprised of State Medicaid Directors) to develop a state consultation and review process for our reports and other materials. State Medicaid and CHIP officials review the Commission's Reports to the Congress before publication.

Budget Estimates: *(b)(10) EXAMINATION OF BUDGET CONSEQUENCES.—Before making any recommendations, MACPAC shall examine the budget consequences of such recommendations, directly or through consultation with appropriate expert entities, and shall submit with any recommendations, a report on the Federal and State-specific budget consequences of the recommendations.*

The MACPAC authorizing statute requires that the Commission examine the federal, as well as state-specific, budget consequences of all recommendations directly or through consultation with various expert entities. The Commission is working to develop an approach to estimate the state-level impacts of recommendations in future reports. MACPAC staff has begun discussions with several state-focused organizations and federal budget offices about a potential role they could play in assisting us with state policy analysis and cost projections, as appropriate. The statutory requirement to evaluate state-level impacts reflects the need for analyses that illustrate the diversity among states and their programs. Federal scorekeepers—the Congressional Budget Office (CBO) and the CMS Office of the Actuary—provide separate budget estimates on federal impacts and are not generally required to provide state-specific estimates of changes in federal Medicaid and CHIP policy.

The Medicare Payment Advisory Commission: (b)(11) CONSULTATION AND COORDINATION WITH MEDPAC.—

(A) IN GENERAL.—MACPAC shall consult with the Medicare Payment Advisory Commission (in this paragraph referred to as 'MedPAC') established under section 1805 in carrying out its duties under this section, as appropriate and particularly with respect to the issues specified in paragraph (2) as they relate to those Medicaid beneficiaries who are dually eligible for Medicaid and the Medicare program under title XVIII, adult Medicaid beneficiaries (who are not dually eligible for Medicare), and beneficiaries under Medicare.

Addressing issues related to individuals dually eligible for Medicare and Medicare is an important element of the Commission's activities. MedPAC is an independent Congressional agency that advises the Congress on issues affecting the Medicare program. The two Commissions have actively collaborated on several policy matters, including dually eligible individuals. The Chairs and Vice-Chairs of both MACPAC and MedPAC have met to discuss and coordinate on policy issues and the Commission has been briefed by MedPAC staff in a public session on dually eligible individuals. Plans are in place for ongoing collaboration and coordination on data and policy issues.

Federal Coordinated Health Care Office: *(b)(13) COORDINATE AND CONSULT WITH THE FEDERAL COORDINATED HEALTH CARE OFFICE.—MACPAC shall coordinate and consult with the Federal Coordinated Health Care Office established under section 2081 of the Patient Protection and Affordable Care Act before making any recommendations regarding dual eligible individuals.*

The Federal Coordinated Health Care Office (Medicare-Medicaid Coordination Office) is a new federal agency within the Centers for Medicare & Medicaid Services (CMS) that focuses on policy issues related to individuals who are dually eligible for both Medicaid and Medicare. The Commission has actively worked with this new office and its Director has briefed the Commission on their priorities and activities. This office is briefed on issues prior to each MACPAC public meeting and there is ongoing collaboration around analytic work and data development.

Additional Consultation Activities

The Commission recognizes that the Medicaid and CHIP programs touch a broad array of public- and private-sector stakeholders, including but not limited to the federal and state governments, and enrollee, provider, industry, and state organizations. Consequently the Commission makes a concerted effort to keep stakeholders well informed about the Commission's research and analytic agenda. These ongoing dialogues inform the Commission's work on the numerous issues that states, the federal government, providers, and enrollees face with respect to the Medicaid and CHIP programs. These interactions are supplemented by comments that stakeholder groups share during the public comment period at the Commission's public meetings as well as comments submitted through our website.

Commission Members and Terms

Diane Rowland, Sc.D., Chair
Washington, DC

David Sundwall, M.D., Vice Chair
Salt Lake City, UT

Term Expires
December 2011

Richard Chambers
Santa Ana, CA

Burton Edelstein, D.D.S., M.P.H.
New York, NY

Denise Henning, C.N.M., M.S.N.
Ft. Myers, FL

Judith Moore
McLean, VA

Robin Smith
Awendaw, SC

David Sundwall, M.D.
Salt Lake City, UT

Term Expires
December 2012

Donna Checkett, M.P.A., M.S.W.
Columbia, MO

Patricia Gabow, M.D.
Denver, CO

Mark Hoyt, F.S.A., M.A.A.A.
Desert Hills, AZ

Patricia Riley, M.S.
Brunswick, ME

Diane Rowland, Sc.D.
Washington, DC

Steven Waldren, M.D., M.S.
Kansas City, MO

Term Expires
December 2013

Sharon Carte, M.H.S.
South Charleston, WV

Andrea Cohen, J.D.
New York, NY

Herman Gray, M.D., M.B.A.
W. Bloomfield, MI

Norma Martinez-Rogers, Ph.D., R.N., F.A.A.N.
San Antonio, TX

Sara Rosenbaum, J.D.
Alexandria, VA

Commissioner Biographies

Sharon L. Carte, M.H.S., is executive director of the West Virginia Children's Health Insurance Program. From 1992 to 1998, Ms. Carte served as the deputy commissioner for the Bureau for Medical Services overseeing West Virginia's Medicaid program. Prior to that she was administrator of several skilled and intermediate care nursing facilities and had also worked as coordinator of Human Resources Development in the West Virginia Department of Health. Ms. Carte's experience included work with senior centers and aging programs throughout the state of West Virginia, and policies related to behavioral health and home and community-based services for mentally disabled populations. She received her Master of Health Science from The Johns Hopkins University.

Richard Chambers is chief executive officer of CalOptima, a County Organized Health System, which provides publicly funded health coverage programs for low-income families, seniors, and persons with disabilities in Orange County, California. CalOptima serves more than 415,000 members through Medicaid, CHIP, and Medicare Advantage Special Needs Plan programs. Before joining CalOptima in 2003, Mr. Chambers spent over 27 years working for the Centers for Medicare & Medicaid Services (CMS). He served as the director of the Family and Children's Health Programs Group, responsible for national policy and operational direction of Medicaid and CHIP. Prior to that, Mr. Chambers served as associate regional administrator for Medicaid in the San Francisco Regional Office and director of the Office of Intergovernmental Affairs in the

Washington, DC office. He received his Bachelor of Arts degree from the University of Virginia.

Donna Checkett, M.P.A., M.S.W., is vice president of State Government Relations at Aetna. Prior to that she was the chief executive officer of Missouri Care, a managed Medicaid health plan owned by University of Missouri-Columbia Health Care, one of the largest safety net hospital systems in the state. For eight years Ms. Checkett served as the director of the Missouri Division of Medical Services (Medicaid), during which time she was the chair of the National Association of State Medicaid Directors and a member of the National Governors Association Medicaid Improvements Working Group. She served as chair of the Advisory Board for the Center for Health Care Strategies, a non-profit health policy resource center dedicated to improving health care quality for low-income children and adults. Ms. Checkett also served as chair of the National Advisory Committee for Covering Kids, a Robert Wood Johnson Foundation program fostering outreach and eligibility simplification efforts for Medicaid and CHIP beneficiaries. She received a Master of Public Administration degree from the University of Missouri-Columbia and a Master of Social Work degree from the University of Texas at Austin.

Andrea Cohen, J.D., is the director of Health Services in the New York City Office of the Mayor, coordinating and implementing strategies to improve public health and health care services including the administration of Medicaid eligibility processes. She serves on the board of the Primary Care Development Corporation and represents the Deputy Mayor for Health and Human Services on the Board of the Health and Hospitals Corporation, the largest public hospital system in the country. From 2005 to 2009, Ms. Cohen was counsel with Manatt, Phelps & Phillips, LLP, where she advised clients on issues relating to Medicare, Medicaid and other public health insurance programs. Prior professional positions include senior policy counsel at the Medicare Rights Center, Health and Oversight Counsel for the U.S. Senate Committee on Finance, and attorney with the U.S. Department of Justice. Ms. Cohen received her law degree from the Columbia University School of Law.

Burton L. Edelstein, D.D.S., M.P.H., is a board-certified pediatric dentist and professor of Dentistry and of Health Policy and Management at Columbia University. He is founding president of the Children's Dental Health Project, a national non-profit policy organization based in Washington, DC, which promotes equity in children's oral health. Dr. Edelstein practiced pediatric dentistry in Connecticut and taught at the Harvard School of Dental Medicine for 21 years prior to serving as a 1996-1997 Robert Wood Johnson Health policy fellow in the office of U.S. Senate minority leader with primary responsibility for S-CHIP. Dr. Edelstein worked with the U.S. Department of Health and Human Services on its oral health initiatives from 1998 to 2001, chaired the U.S. Surgeon General's Workshop on Children and Oral Health, and authored the child section of Oral Health in America: A Report of the Surgeon General. His research focuses on children's oral health promotion and access to dental care with a particular emphasis on Medicaid and CHIP populations. Dr. Edelstein received his degree in dentistry from the State University of New York at Buffalo School of Dentistry, his Master of Public Health degree from the Harvard School of Public Health, and completed his clinical training at Children's Hospital Boston.

Patricia Gabow, M.D., is chief executive officer of Denver Health and Hospital Authority, an integrated public safety-net health care system that is the state's largest provider of care to Medicaid and uninsured patients. Dr. Gabow is a member of the Commonwealth Fund's Commission on a High-Performing Health System and previously served as chair of the National Association of Public Hospitals. She also served on Institute of Medicine committees, including one that addressed the future viability of safety-net providers and another that addressed performance measures and quality improvement. Dr. Gabow joined Denver Health in 1973 as chief of the Renal Division and is a professor of Medicine in the Division of Renal Diseases at the University of Colorado Denver School of Medicine. She received her medical degree from the University of Pennsylvania.

Herman Gray, M.D., M.B.A., is president of the Children's Hospital of Michigan and senior vice president of the Detroit Medical Center, having served in these roles since 2005. Previously, at the Children's Hospital of Michigan, Dr. Gray served as chief operating officer, chief of staff, pediatric residency program director, and pediatrics vice chief for education. He also held positions as associate dean for graduate medical education at Wayne State University School of Medicine and vice president for Graduate Medical Education (GME) at the Detroit Medical Center. In the 1990s, Dr. Gray was the chief medical consultant (medical director) for the Michigan Department of Public Health – Children's Special Health Care Services, and later became vice president and medical director of Clinical Affairs for Blue Care Network, a 600,000 member subsidiary of Blue Cross/Blue Shield of Michigan. During the 1980s, he pursued private medical practice in Detroit while acting as a member of the academic faculty at the Children's Hospital of Michigan and Wayne State University. Dr. Gray currently chairs the Detroit Medical Center GME Work Group and serves on the board of trustees of the National Association of Children's Hospitals and Related Institutions, the board of directors of the Child Health Corporation of America, and the American Hospital Association Section for Maternal and Child Health Governing Council. Dr. Gray was named in 2010 as a Top 25 Minority Executive in Healthcare by Modern Healthcare Magazine. He received his medical degree from the University of Michigan in Ann Arbor and an executive Master of Business Administration from the University of Tennessee.

Denise Henning, C.N.M., M.S.N., is a clinical director for women's health at Collier Health Services, a federally qualified health center in Immokalee, Florida. A practicing nurse-midwife, Ms. Henning provides prenatal and gynecological care to a service population that is predominantly either uninsured or covered by Medicaid. From 2003 to 2008 she was director of Clinical Operations for Women's Health Services at the Family Health Centers of Southwest Florida, where she supervised midwifery and other clinical staff. Prior to this, Ms. Henning served as a Certified Nurse Midwife in several locations in Florida and as a labor and delivery nurse in a Level III teaching hospital. She is president of the Midwifery Business Network and a chapter chair of the American College of Nurse Midwives. Ms. Henning received her Master of Science degree in Nurse-Midwifery from the University of Florida in Jacksonville and her Bachelor of Science in Nursing from the University of Florida in Gainesville.

Mark Hoyt, F.S.A., M.A.A.A., is a senior partner with the Government Human Services Consulting group of Mercer Health & Benefits LLC. The Government specialty group focuses on helping states become more efficient purchasers of Medicaid and CHIP health services and has worked with more than 30 states. Mr. Hoyt joined Mercer in 1980 and since 1987 has worked on government health care projects, including developing strategies for statewide health reform, evaluating the impact of different managed care approaches, and overseeing program design and rate analyses for Medicaid and CHIP programs. Mr. Hoyt is a fellow in the Society of Actuaries and a member of the American Academy of Actuaries. He received a Master of Arts degree in mathematics from the University of California at Berkeley.

Norma Martinez Rogers, Ph.D., R.N., F.A.A.N., is professor of the Department of Family Nursing at the University of Texas Health Science Center at San Antonio, where she has served on the faculty since 1996. Dr. Martinez Rogers has held clinical and administrative positions in psychiatric nursing and psychiatric hospitals, including the William Beaumont Army Medical Center in Fort Bliss during Operation Desert Storm. She has initiated a number of programs at the University of Texas Health Science Center in San Antonio including a support group for women transitioning from prison back into society and the Martinez Street Women's Center, a non-profit organization designed to provide support and educational services to women and teenage girls. Dr. Martinez Rogers is a fellow of the American Academy of Nursing and is president of the National Association of Hispanic Nurses. She received a Master of Science degree in Psychiatric Nursing from the University of Texas Health Science Center at San Antonio and a Doctor of Philosophy degree in Cultural Foundations in Education from the University of Texas at Austin. She was recently selected by the National Diversity Council as one of 20 women who are considered to be the most influential and powerful women in Texas.

Judith Moore is senior fellow at the National Health Policy Forum, George Washington University, where she specializes in work related to the health needs of low-income vulnerable populations. Prior to joining the Forum, Ms. Moore held positions in both the legislative and executive branches of the federal government. At the Health Care Financing Administration (now the Centers for Medicare & Medicaid Services), she directed the Medicaid program and the Office of Legislation and Congressional Affairs. Ms. Moore was special assistant to the Secretary of the Department of Health, Education and Welfare (now the Department of Health and Human Services) and held positions in the Public Health Service, the Food and Drug Administration, the Agency for Health Care Policy and Research, and the Prospective Payment Assessment Commission. She is co-author of a political history of Medicaid, Medicaid Politics and Policy, 1965-2007.

Trish Riley, M.S., is the first distinguished visiting fellow and lecturer in State Health Policy at George Washington University, following her tenure as director of the Maine Governor's Office of Health Policy and Finance. She was a principal architect of the Dirigo Health Reform Act of 2003, which was enacted to increase access, reduce costs, and improve quality of health care in Maine. Ms. Riley previously served as executive director of the National Academy for State Health Policy and as president of its Corporate Board. Under four Maine governors, she held appointed positions including executive director of the Maine Committee on Aging; director of the Bureau of Maine's Elderly; associate deputy commissioner of Health and Medical Services; and director of the Bureau of Medical Services, the Medicaid agency, that also included licensure and certification and health planning. Ms. Riley served on Maine's Commission on Children's Health, which planned the state's SCHIP program. She is a member of the Kaiser Commission on Medicaid

and the Uninsured and has served as a member of the Institute of Medicine's Subcommittee on Creating an External Environment for Quality and its Subcommittee on Maximizing the Value of Health. Ms. Riley has also served as a member of the Board of Directors of the National Committee on Quality Assurance. She received her Master of Science degree in Community Development from the University of Maine.

Sara Rosenbaum, J.D., is the Harold and Jane Hirsh Professor and Founding Chair of the Department of Health Policy, George Washington University School of Public Health and Health Services, a unique center of learning, scholarship, and public service focusing on all aspects of health policy. Professor Rosenbaum has devoted her career to issues of health law and policy affecting low income, minority, and medically underserved populations. Between 1993 and 1994, Professor Rosenbaum worked for President Clinton, directing the legislative drafting of the Health Security Act and developing the Vaccines for Children program. Professor Rosenbaum also served on the Presidential Transition Team for President-Elect Obama. A graduate of Wesleyan University and Boston University School of Law, Professor Rosenbaum has authored a leading health law textbook as well as more than 350 articles and studies focusing on all phases of health law and health care for medically underserved populations. A holder of numerous awards for her scholarship and service, Professor Rosenbaum is the recipient of the Richard and Barbara Hansen National Health Leadership Award (University of Iowa), a Robert Wood Johnson Foundation Investigator Award in Health Policy Research, and the Oscar and Shoshanna Trachtenberg Award for scholarship (George Washington University's highest award for scholarship). Professor Rosenbaum is a member of Center for Disease Control and Prevention's Advisory Committee on Immunization Practice (ACIP) and Director's Advisory Committee.

Diane Rowland, Sc.D., is the executive vice president of the Henry J. Kaiser Family Foundation and the executive director of the Kaiser Commission on Medicaid and the Uninsured. She is also an adjunct professor in the Department of Health Policy and Management at the Bloomberg School of Public Health of the Johns Hopkins University. She has directed the Kaiser Commission since 1991 and overseen the Foundation's health policy work since 1993. She is a noted authority on health policy, Medicare and Medicaid, and health care for low-income and disadvantaged populations, and frequently testifies as an expert witness before the U.S. Congress on health policy issues. A nationally recognized expert with a distinguished career in public policy and research focusing on health insurance coverage, access to care, and health care financing, Dr. Rowland is an accomplished researcher and has published widely on these subjects. Dr. Rowland is a member of the IOM, a founding member of the National Academy for Social Insurance, past president and fellow of the Association for Health Services Research (now AcademyHealth), and a member of the board of Grantmakers in Health. She holds a Bachelor's degree from Wellesley College, a Master of Public Administration from the University of California at Los Angeles and a Doctor of Science degree in health policy and management from the Johns Hopkins University. Dr. Rowland serves as chair of MACPAC.

Robin Smith and her husband Doug have been foster and adoptive parents for children covered by Medicaid, including many special needs children. Her experience with the health care system includes the Medically Fragile Children's Program, an interdisciplinary Medicaid program at the Medical University of South Carolina Children's Hospital, which is a national model partnership between MUSC Children's Hospital, South Carolina Medicaid and the South Carolina Department of Social Services. Ms. Smith serves on the Family Advisory Committee for the Children's Hospital at the Medical University of South Carolina. She has testified at Congressional briefings, presented at the 2007 International Conference of Family Centered Care, and participated in Grand Rounds for medical students and residents at the Medical University of South Carolina. In November 2010 she was awarded the Health Care Hero Award by the Charleston Regional Business Journal.

David Sundwall, M.D., is a professor of Public Health at the University of Utah School of Medicine, Division of Public Health, where he has been a faculty member since 1978. He served as executive director of the Utah Department of Health and commissioner of Health for the State of Utah, from 2005 through 2010. He currently serves on numerous government and community boards and advisory groups in his home state, including serving as chair of the State Controlled Substance Advisory Committee. He also serves as vice chair of the federal Medicaid and CHIP Payment and Access Commission [MACPAC] in Washington, DC. Dr. Sundwall served as president of the Association of State and Territorial Health Officials (ASTHO) from 2007-08. He has chaired or served on several committees of the Institute of Medicine (IOM) – currently on the Committee on Integration of Primary Care and Public Health, and the Standing Committee on Health Threats Resilience. Prior to returning to Utah in 2005, he was president of the American Clinical Laboratory Association (ACLA) and prior to that was vice president and Medical Director of American Healthcare Systems (AmHS). Dr. Sundwall's federal government experience includes serving as administrator of the Health Resources and Services Administration (HRSA), assistant surgeon general in the Commissioned Corps of the U.S. Public Health Service, and director of the Health and Human Resources Staff of the Senate Labor and Human Resources Committee. He received his medical degree from the University of Utah

School of Medicine, and completed residency in the Harvard Family Medicine Program. He is a licensed physician, board certified in Internal Medicine and Family Practice, and volunteers in a public health clinic one-half day each week.

Steven E. Waldren, M.D., M.S., joined the American Academy of Family Physicians (AAFP) in 2004 and serves as director of its Center for Health Information Technology. His in-depth knowledge of health information systems, programming and software, and medical informatics makes him a qualified expert to lead the Center as it aims to expand its services to thousands more primary care physicians. Dr. Waldren also serves on the board of the Center for Improving Medication Management, a national advocacy organization that educates clinicians and their staff on the best approaches to implementing prescribing technology. He also serves as co-chair of the Ambulatory Care Quality Alliance's Data Aggregation and Health IT Subcommittee. Dr. Waldren earned a master's degree in health care informatics from the University of Missouri, Columbia, while completing a National Library of Medicine Postdoctoral Medical Informatics Research Fellowship. He completed his family medicine residency at Wesley Family Medicine in Wichita, Kansas, and earned his medical degree from the University of Kansas School of Medicine, Kansas City.

Commission Staff

Lu Zawistowich, Sc.D.
Executive Director

Office of the Executive Director

Patti Barnett, M.Sc.
Michelle Herman, M.H.S.
Linda Mac Nally
Mary Ellen Stahlman, M.H.S.A.

Analytic Staff

April Grady, M.P.Aff.
Caroline Haarmann, M.P.H.
Molly McGinn-Shapiro, M.P.P.
Christie Peters, M.P.P.
Chris Peterson, M.P.P.
Lois Simon, M.H.S.
James Teisl, M.P.H.
Jennifer Tracey, M.H.A.

Operations and Management

Libbie Buchele, M.P.P., M.P.H.
Chief Operating Officer

Mathew Chase
Chief Information Officer

Research Assistant

Dominique Hodo

www.ingramcontent.com/pod-product-compliance
Lightning Source LLC
Chambersburg PA
CBHW081114170526
45165CB00008B/2445